Who will I be when I die?

Who will
I be when
I die?

Christine Bryden

Foreword by Elizabeth MacKinlay

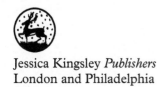

Jessica Kingsley *Publishers*
London and Philadelphia

Published in 2012
by Jessica Kingsley Publishers
73 Collier Street
London N1 9BE, UK
and
400 Market Street, Suite 400
Philadelphia, PA 19106, USA

www.jkp.com

First published in 1998 by HarperCollinsReligious,
an imprint of HarperCollins, Australia

Library of Congress Cataloging in Publication Data
A CIP catalog record for this book is available from the Library of Congress

British Library Cataloguing in Publication Data
A CIP catalogue record for this book is available from the British Library

ISBN 978 1 84905 312 9
eISBN 978 0 85700 645 5

Printed and bound in Great Britain

Dedication

To my second husband, Paul, who enables me to keep doing my best, despite my daily struggle to cope. We met in 1998, a few months after this book was first published. With him beside me, encouraging and supporting me, I have lasted far longer than anyone would have dreamed possible. I know he will be there when I have lost so much more, and he will still love me for my inner self.

To my three delightful daughters who love me unconditionally, despite my quirky functioning and changing needs. Once, long ago, I was their busy, career-driven mother. Now I am slower and more dependent, but still I can marvel at their achievements and delight in their happiness. My hope is that as I decline even further, they will keep on loving me for who I am, without any pity or sorrow in their eyes for the loss of who I once was.

Contents

Foreword

It is an honour to write a foreword to this republished edition of Christine Bryden's first book. Christine is a remarkable woman of great courage and strength. I first met her shortly before her diagnosis of dementia was confirmed. When I accepted Christine's invitation to journey with her into this disease as both geriatric nurse and priest, I could never have guessed how life changing this would be for me, quite apart from the primary and intended purpose of supporting Christine. As I journeyed with her, I realised that much more was possible for people with dementia than was often supposed and I strongly encouraged Christine to write this book. Meeting regularly with Christine I found, for the first time, I was able to hear from a person who has dementia what it felt like to experience this disease.

Christine found herself, as a young woman, suddenly cast into a new and unwanted role in life. From the time of her diagnosis, Christine has pushed boundaries of the expected symptoms of this disease; she has not ceased to push boundaries. She has been a strong advocate for others with dementia and she has lived her life since diagnosis with faith, courage and tenacity. It has been a privilege to journey with Christine, as she experienced and challenged the changes that this disease brought, and to witness her continuing faith in the face of dementia.

A common stereotype is that people with dementia can't speak and interact normally with others. The very fact that Christine was able to express herself in writing and speaking meant her diagnosis was discounted by numbers of people. The stereotypes of dementia, be it Alzheimer's disease, vascular dementia, or one of the other dementias, make it difficult for people with dementia and those who care for them to live satisfying lives of meaning. It was Christine who challenged me to study where people with dementia find meaning. Fear still surrounds this disease, and yet there is hope, right in the midst of this disease, not just for a cure, but in finding new ways to live faithfully with this disease, to challenge it and overcome stigma and exclusion that still exist in many places.

There are more books written by the families of those who have dementia than are written by people who have dementia. I am delighted that this book of a first-hand account of dementia is being republished. I know it has been inspirational for many who have dementia and for their families. These days, most people say that they know someone who has dementia, and it is my hope that Christine's words will be read by many others, who will also find inspiration in her journey, her strength and her faith, which have carried her through all this time. Yes, her story is studded with hope and joys, large and small. Her story also contains sadness and great challenges. I highly recommend this book to people who have this disease, their carers, health professionals and the wider community; indeed, to all who may be touched in any way with Alzheimer's disease, or any other type of dementia.

Elizabeth MacKinlay
January 2012
Canberra

Memories of Christine

What do I see as being different between the 'now' Christine and the 'then' Christine? The main difference is speed – she certainly doesn't juggle projects and ideas like she used to. We still share memories, and have very astute conversations about governments, politics, and other people's decisions. She is much more sensitive to people's feelings than she used to be, and much more passive – someone else does the organising. The 'now' Christine is slower, sometimes forgets the names of things, takes longer to understand new information and may not remember what I have told her (for example, names of plants). While the doctors may tell her she has lost a lot of brain function, they don't realise how much she had to start with – so losing some brain cells has brought her back to less than average, from stratospherically high. A lot of people ask after her when I say I have been in touch, but none of them ever contact her directly – too scared I suppose, not knowing what they will find. However, I am glad that our friendship has been able to continue and hope that it will continue that way for a long time to come.

Dr Lyndal Thorburn
Viria Pty Ltd (work collegue, mid-1980s to mid-1990s)

Preface

The present day

My journey with dementia has been an unexpectedly long one – from the time of diagnosis in 1995, described in this book, to sixteen years of gradual decline, so that now my former self has become unrecognisable. That high-powered, cool, calm and collected person has become lost and forgotten along the way. Now I am slow, emotionally unpredictable and confused in a maze of words, numbers and endless 'thingys'.

At the beginning of this journey I was paralysed by fear – 'Who will I be when I die?' Could I fight this disease with dignity and strength, or would these characteristics of inner fortitude be eaten away by the disease process? Writing this book was a way of reflecting on my fears, of discovering reserves of courage, and finding in my Christian faith and fellowship a way to look to the future with hope.

I looked for precious moments with my daughters and in the garden, as I found an inner peace. I felt reassured that what I was losing was my outer masks of cognition and emotion, while my true inner self remained. This realisation came a few years into my journey with dementia, while I was writing my second book, *Dancing with Dementia* (2005).

The original publication of this first book, in 1998, saw the beginning of my efforts in advocacy. At that time, diagnosis meant a presumption of being unable to speak – of being 'a mindless, empty shell'. There was a lack of support and inclusion for people with dementia, which inspired me to become a passionate advocate for the millions of people around the world who can no longer speak. I talk about these efforts in my second book, but it is this first book that marked the beginning of this new life of advocacy.

But how could I do any of this, with my inability to cope with stress, to find my way, to organise or plan, or to think clearly? The year this book was first published was also the beginning of a new life with my second husband, Paul. He has been my enabler, helping me to achieve despite my many limitations. We have travelled extensively and made many friends in the worldwide Alzheimer's movement.

I am so grateful that people all around the world have listened, and changed their views. Now people with dementia are receiving much better support to help them cope with declining brain function. But still there are no cures for the many diseases, including Alzheimer's, that cause dementia. Dementia is the third biggest killer in the developed world. Why is there so little effort in finding cures? Is it because we think it's a normal part of ageing, or because we fear it so much? But it's not a normal part of ageing – only one in four people over the age of 80 are likely to develop dementia – my grandmother was 108 years old when she died, and showed no signs of any dementia. We need to regard these diseases as the killers that they are, and urgently to seek cures. Already there are nearly 36 million people around the world dying from dementia. We are told cures are maybe at least twenty years away, by which time there will be over 65 million people with dementia, escalating to over 115 million by 2050.

For me, since 1998, life has continued to be a roller-coaster ride of ups and downs. There have been many memorable moments – a beautiful day for my daughter's wedding to a lovely young man, delightful times with my two grandchildren, and a wonderful ceremony for my daughter's graduation. Each of these was an experience that I never expected to live to see when I wrote this book. Other highs include receiving a standing ovation for the first presentation by a person with dementia at the Alzheimer's Disease International conference in 2001, and being elected to its Board in 2003. But there have been some very low points on the home front, when I was unable to cope adequately with the stress and anxiety of my daughters as they came to terms with my decline. And in my advocacy, there were other lows. I faced huge challenges to my credibility because I could still speak, and even had my brain scans questioned because of my level of function. Without Paul alongside me, to pick up the pieces and to encourage me to continue despite these attacks on my honesty and integrity, I could not have kept up the pace of advocacy for change. There have also been so many emails encouraging me, telling me how much my books have helped both those with dementia and those caring for them. These have often come at low times when I needed to be uplifted and inspired to keep going.

As I reflect on the journey since this first book was published in 1998, I feel so very blessed to have my loving husband, Paul, by my side, and my three daughters living happily with their partners. Ianthe is now thirty-seven and has an excellent job as a physiotherapist in a large hospital, balancing this with life at home with her partner and two lively and delightful children. Rhiannon is now thirty-one and married, with a very rewarding job coordinating hospital improvements in our region, while at home her passion is fulfilled, with horses on acreage. Micheline is now twenty-six and has graduated with a first-class honours degree in history and is well on track to succeeding in her dream career in academia, balanced by a happy home life with her partner.

For me, I will do my best, with Paul's help, to continue advocacy – to speak out for all of those who either cannot speak or don't want to speak about this feared fatal disease.

Christine Bryden
November 2011

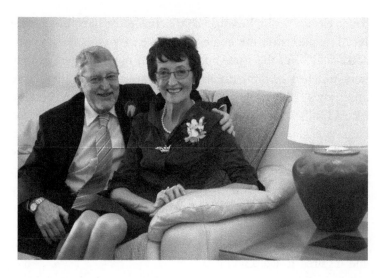

Paul and Christine, September 2009, ready to go to Rhiannon's wedding

Fourteen years ago

My life has undergone a dramatic change, with a strong impact on me and my three daughters: in the space of a few days in 1995 I changed from being a busy senior executive/sole parent, with a successful career, to being a pensioner (and still a single mum) with a limited life expectancy.

I was diagnosed in May 1995, at the age of only forty-six, with the early stages of Alzheimer's disease, and then spent six months seeking a second opinion from another neurologist, undergoing every possible test. The diagnosis was confirmed.

It's not certain how quickly the disease will progress, but maybe I'll need some assistance with personal care soon, and maybe full nursing care within a few years. The material I have read points to life expectancies that can be as short as about six to eight years after symptoms first become quite obvious. But I have experienced a miraculous improvement in my functioning, which I describe in the postscript – so I will ignore statistics and medical expectations and enjoy the life given to me!

I have no regrets about my life – and have crammed a wealth of experiences into my forty-nine years. The last seven years, since becoming a Christian, have been especially eventful, and indeed it's been like riding God's roller-coaster. No sooner am I settled and enjoying coasting along, when along comes yet another dip and turn in my life. I've held onto my faith in God a bit like the roller-coaster cart hangs onto the rails!

I am writing down my memories for my daughters, Ianthe, Rhiannon and Micheline, who are now aged twenty-three, seventeen and twelve, as I am very much aware that a biological deadline could be rapidly approaching, when I can no longer read or write. I want them to know about some of my life's experiences, before I am no longer able to communicate them. As part of this, I have written this book about my emotional, physical and spiritual journey with Alzheimer's disease. I know that it, somehow, is part of God's purpose in my life – so much so that I think of it as 'God's book', not Christine's book. But when I sat down to start, I had no idea what I would actually say – apart from the fact that without my faith in God, I would not have been able to cope with this devastating illness.

There are many misconceptions about the disease, including: you don't die from it; it only afflicts old people; you simply become a bit doddery and forgetful; it's just losing your memory. It is, however, the fourth most common cause of death in Australia, 2 per cent of cases are early-onset (that is, occur in people under the age of sixty-five; I'm just forty-nine), life expectancy can be about eight years from diagnosis, and you slowly lose the ability to know how to do things (such as operate a stove, drive a car and so on), until eventually you even forget how to run your body (many patients die choking on their food because they no longer know how to swallow).

I've briefly described Alzheimer's disease, as well as giving insights into its various stages, in Appendix I. I want to expose the myths, make clear what it is – and isn't. It is one of the most poorly understood terminal illnesses in our society, although it affects so many of us – and the number of cases will escalate dramatically as the 'baby-boomers' begin to succumb. With more information, I hope some people may get diagnosed earlier, and that they and their families can be helped to understand and cope with this disease that robs you of much of what makes you who you are.

There are not many books written by Alzheimer's sufferers, as generally they tend not to be aware of their gradual deterioration, nor to be able to document the changes happening to them. There are several written by carers, which have a very different perspective.

Each Alzheimer's sufferer has slightly different experiences, as their brain slowly disappears, and I was 'lucky' to be diagnosed early enough to leave work before I began to make serious errors. I was sent for some routine scans to check whether my frequent migraines had a physical cause. In a way they did: the migraine attacks were triggered by coping with my job as First Assistant Secretary in the Department of Prime Minister and Cabinet (a position two steps from the head of a department), as well as the emotional trauma and financial strain of leaving my husband in early 1993, while my brain was slowly wasting away. Although in 1991 I had graduated with a Master of Business Administration, and in 1992 was featured in a Public Service Commission book on six women and their careers, by the time I was awarded the Public Service medal for outstanding service to science and technology, in the Queen's Birthday Honours List in 1994, my brain cells were becoming fewer and fewer, and the early signs of the disease were there.

My book is not a miserable story. I am happy and very much at peace with what is happening to me. My life has been challenging and interesting. I have three delightful daughters – each a totally different and fascinating individual in her own right. I have also enjoyed an interesting career in Europe and Australia. Starting off in scientific research, then publishing, I moved to a large science organisation and was involved in setting up a space science program, as well as in the 'business' of research for the minerals industry. I then became a senior bureaucrat in

science and technology, and gave advice to government, ran a
large funding program, and involved ministers more actively
in understanding the potential of Australian research and
application.

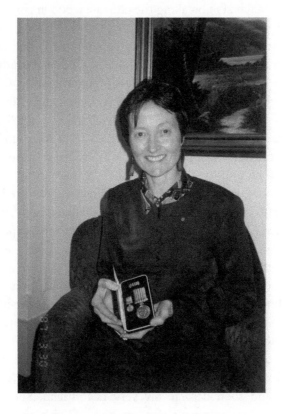

Public Service Medal award September 1994

All of this variety, this fun, this learning and doing, has made
me a bit of a trailblazer perhaps. At any rate, I am determined to
attack this Alzheimer's disease with the same vigour that I put
into my work and my girls. Alzheimer's is a bit of a taboo subject
– or a bit of a joke. Families of sufferers are often ashamed of
their very odd, 'batty' relative, and can't understand why they
can't stop this silly behaviour. I am hoping to break that taboo –

of being ashamed of a disease. Why be ashamed of the physical breakdown of brain cells any more than the physical breakdown of other parts of our body? We are not mad, but sick, so please treat us with dignity, do not make fun of us, and do not be ashamed. Maybe I'm breaking the ultimate taboo in going public and saying 'I have dementia!'

Christianity, too, is a bit of a secret topic – you are not meant to talk openly about your faith in God, apparently. This seems to be no longer 'acceptable' in countries like Australia. Well, God gets lots of mention in this book – my faith is part of my life, in all the ordinary bits as well as the more 'holy' or traumatic bits – and if this offends, then I am sorry, and hope that you can somehow skip those 'God-bits' to read about more 'normal' topics.

This book could not have been written without the help of many people. Ianthe, Rhiannon and Micheline deserve the first vote of thanks. They are sharing with you, the reader, experiences which even now cause them pain, suffering and grief and may continue to do so, if this disease robs them of their mother and best friend bit by bit, day by day. But I commit them now to God, who will take care of them and surround them with love, support and friendship through any journey they must make along with me.

First of all I'd like to thank Margaret Frisch. She was my personal assistant at the Department of Prime Minister and Cabinet, and soon became my very dear friend. She was an amazing source of support for me and my girls through the trauma of the first few months, looking after the girls when I was in Sydney for tests, and with phone calls, cards, flowers and visits letting us know that caring help was never far away. It was some months before the results were certain, and in this period – the time of fear, confusion and disbelief – Margaret was our lifeline.

After the results were confirmed, I finally felt able to share with my church, St George's Anglican Life Centre, Canberra. The prayers, practical help, love and understanding of the whole congregation have been one of the greatest blessings that

God could give me and my girls. Particular thanks must go to Christine Morrissey and Clare Reeves, who organised practical and prayerful support to my family, and to Chris and Kathryn Simon, our rector and his wife, who provided teaching, love and encouragement, and who faithfully prayed with me through several crises in my life.

Many others at St George's have prayed, made meals, driven my girls to various venues – there are too many to name individually – to them all, I offer my heartfelt thanks for being my loving family-in-Christ who have made writing this book a possibility.

This book would probably never have been finished, or published, without Liz MacKinlay, my 'spiritual director' – this word is 'Anglican-speak' for someone I meet regularly with to talk to about God, and who helps me, advises me, comforts me. She has given me much encouragement, advice and reassurance, when I have felt like giving up, or simply been so discouraged by the size of the task and the difficulty of writing in any detail. She is an assistant priest at Cooma, chaplain of the University of Canberra, a wife and a mother, a specialist lecturer in gerontological nursing…and somehow she managed to find the time to meet with me, to read my attempts at writing, to pray with me, to offer advice, and most of all to encourage me.

Jeffi Hill, the librarian at the Alzheimer's Association of NSW, has also been an important part of making this book a reality. Not only did she provide excellent information about the disease, but she has also encouraged me in sharing our faith. I first met her through her husband, when he and I were studying for our Master of Business Administration, long before I had any inkling of what was happening inside my head.

Other friends, too, have been encouraging, supporting me in prayer, and in letters. My best friend in Sydney, Karen Stott, and her husband Roger, are my friends for eternity, through all of life's experiences – through their own experiences of cancer and chronic fatigue syndrome and through my Alzheimer's disease – they love, pray for and support me, and I know my girls will have such love to turn to if I can no longer be there for them. It is through Karen that I became a Christian.

I owe a special debt to my family – my mother and father, my aunt and grandmother – who have been my inspiration to succeed, to experience, and to enjoy. They gave me and my sister the gift no-one else could possibly have offered – a happy and carefree childhood. Their love, generosity and support now, albeit from a distance, is giving me great comfort, and in so many ways they have shown me often just how much they care, although they live half a world away, in England and in Belgium.

My grandmother turned 103 this year, and is still at home, cooking, in charge, and very much alert and interested in life. Her serenity and her quiet no-nonsense faith have been a backdrop to my sometimes chaotic life, and I hope to show maybe just a glimpse of this serenity in the few years left to me.

There are always far too many people to mention, and I feel overwhelmed by the wonderful friends and family that I have.

How could I possibly ever complain that my life has not been a full and happy one? And now I have God on my side too – so my life continues for ever, in great happiness. How could anyone want for more?

Christine Bryden
April 1998

The diagnosis

I'm too young!

The neurologist with his back towards me, looking at my scans, said, 'Your brain is like that of a much older person, showing signs of marked atrophy, particularly at the front. It's consistent with Alzheimer's.'

He looked away from the scans for a moment, and then said, 'You shouldn't be in any responsible position. You must retire as soon as possible.'

I felt as if time had stood still – surely this wasn't happening to me. I had to rush away in a minute and chair a meeting back at work, and I had moved house over the weekend and was still unpacking and sorting out.

I must have misheard – he was mistaken – the scans maybe had got mixed up with someone else's... 'You're joking – I'm too young to get Alzheimer's!'

I was only forty-six – old by my daughters' reckoning, but surely far too young to get an old people's disease like Alzheimer's. Any rate, I wasn't forgetful, just stressed out – with migraines and getting a little confused every now and then – taking the wrong turn a few times surely didn't mean I was getting senile!

The specialist sat down, leaning back on his chair with his hands behind his head and, with what seemed like almost a touch of pride in his voice, he said: 'I've diagnosed a young mother of thirty with Alzheimer's. I've seen diplomats, lawyers, judges retire for the same reason. You really must take action now to retire on medical grounds.'

His bow tie caught my attention – jauntily poised above his crisp white chest. I needed something to focus on, something real to make sure this wasn't all a dream. It was neatly tied, not a clip-on, I was sure, and had quite a subtle pattern for something as ostentatious as a bow tie.

He glanced at the scans again. 'It is not likely to be Pick's, as the loss would then be all in the frontal lobes, and although you've got damage there, you've also got generalised atrophy all through, and enlarged ventricles at the centre. I'd like you to have psychometric tests done soon, too.'

'Er…how long will it be before I…er…um …' I stuttered.

'Until you become demented? Oh, about five years I expect,' answered the specialist, breezily.

The world seemed quite unreal as I walked to my car, as if I were in a dream and soon would wake up to my normal busy life of working in the office and at home every day of the week – fitting in my three girls, shopping, cooking, cleaning, in between. Being a single mum certainly was stressful, and I had just taken out a six-figure mortgage to buy a townhouse – and we had just moved in that weekend.

It was a crystal-clear, crisp autumn Monday morning. The sky was a deep blue, with just a few powdery clouds adrift high above. The trees were showing their beautiful autumn copper-bronzes and eucalypt grey-greens. The sky was huge – stretched out across Canberra and etched around with the soft blue-green mountain ranges in the hazy distance. How could all this beauty exist out here, when all was turmoil inside my head?

My mortgage – what would happen if I retired? Could I still afford it? This had all happened too soon after taking out the mortgage for my insurance to be valid! This at least was a concrete thing to work on. Yes, my first stop had to be the credit union. I drove around the calm deep blue lake, fringed with trembling golden poplars, and drank in the scenery as a balm to calm my mounting anxiety. The credit union manager was kind and helpful, seeing my tension and responding to my need. He took all the details, and offered to help in any way, such as in any financial advice I might need.

I walked back outside into the sunshine, getting into the car and filling my mind with the relative security of today's work schedule. I drove to the office with only a few moments to spare before walking into the conference room to chair an important meeting. I felt remote from proceedings, struggling to keep focused on the task at hand, and getting the outcomes we had sought.

Margaret, my personal assistant and friend, was a tower of strength. She came into my office, after the meeting, shutting the door behind her. 'How did it go at the doctor today?' Tears welled up in her eyes as I told her, but we both struggled to keep our emotions under control, as we had a lot of immediate actions to take. I was obviously in no fit state to cope, and would be seeing my family doctor later that day. I needed to be freed up from as much as possible over the next few days, so that I could have meetings with personnel, senior staff and with the head of our department. The reactions at each of these meetings were similar – disbelief, overwhelming concern and tremendous support.

My family doctor was very concerned, when I saw her that afternoon. She was appalled at the callous attitude of the specialist, and clearly very concerned for me. She got on the phone while I was in her surgery, and managed to get me in to see a specialist in Sydney in eight days' time, to seek a second opinion. She firmly recommended that I not drive there from Canberra, and that I should take immediate sick leave for three weeks. For once in my life I agreed to some time off work. I needed some space to deal with all this.

Those eight days were a nightmare, but at least I had a complete household of boxes to sort out after our move. I unpacked boxes, moved furniture, put up pictures, cleaned... anything to avoid thinking. Even my prayers were confused, clutching for God as a drowning man might desperately fumble around for driftwood. But unlike driftwood, God was – and is – a rock and a tower of strength.

I asked my friends Maureen and Clare to pray for me, and invited Maureen, who had been my neighbour years ago in Sydney (before either of us had become Christians, and while both of us were trying to maintain the public appearance of a normal marriage while we both were being abused by our husbands behind closed doors), to travel with me on the bus to Sydney.

I arranged to see my rector, Chris, and his wife, Kathryn (a nurse) and appeared at their door on a crisply cold dark evening, armed with scans, with an absolute conviction that whatever was going to come out of all this, it would be to God's glory. I sank into their blissfully comfortable easy chair, and talked. They listened, and then prayed. To my surprise and delight, Chris anointed me with oil – not a liquid cooking oil, as I had imagined, but a delicately fragrant ointment out of a tiny screw-top jar.

I drove from their house – even delighting in the colours of the traffic lights, and almost tasting the beauty of the clear dark sky, lit with stars and a tiny piece of moon. I was singing at the top of my voice, and my spiritual and emotional batteries had been charged up enough to last me the next few days up to the bus trip.

I felt physically sick, very tired and strung out, but the four-hour bus journey was a wonderful time of sharing with Maureen, who prayed and talked about where God was in all this. I left her at the bus station, and trundled my bag a few blocks up the hill to the hospital, where the specialist had arranged for me to have further tests and nuclear scans.

Lying on the scanning table I was emotionally drained and exhausted – it was probably one of the lowest points in my life, for despite its ups and downs, life had never before or since struck me down quite as low as this.

As I lay there, with the machine slowly clicking its way around my head, I had a powerful image – that I was not lying on the cold steel table but on a lush field of green soft grass, bathed in warm sunshine from above. But then as I looked closer, zooming in, each blade of grass came into view – the grass was made up of the uplifted fingers of all those praying for me. I quietly thanked God for the peace that this gave me.

After the scans, I trundled my bags back down the hill to Sydney's central station and took a train to the suburbs. This area was my old stamping ground, and I felt comfortable amongst the familiar bustle of the streets of central Sydney. My eldest daughter, Ianthe, who was studying first-year Physiotherapy at the University of Sydney, met me at the train station and drove me back to her group house.

She sat me on her bed and brought me a plate of delicious pancakes, topped with creamy butter, fine sugar and cinnamon. Later that evening she uncorked a small bottle of rainforest-scented massage oil, and gently eased away the tensions so that I drifted into a peaceful and deep sleep – the first since the diagnosis.

I felt decidedly strengthened the next day, as we went back to the hospital for more tests and to meet with the new specialist.

What a difference this quietly spoken and immaculately groomed specialist was to make to my spirits. No irritating bow tie, but wearing a modest silver-coloured tie with a dark blue suit, he sat behind a desk in a small but comfortable office, listening, asking, rather than expressing immediate opinions and statements. He had examined all the results carefully and said it was too early to make a specific diagnosis, and that there were a number of curable diseases to be ruled out before accepting that I had early-onset Alzheimer's.

'You'll need to have a psychometric test, but that's best done when you are less stressed, perhaps in a few months' time. In the meantime we need to get your migraines under control. It's wrong for you to have to take such dangerous drugs simply to be able to continue to work. I recommend you take six months off work while we do further tests.'

Six months! I had hardly ever taken sick leave. I was never sick – or at least never admitted to any illness. I always turned up to work unless I simply was too sick to get out of bed. I'd gone to work with migraines, avoiding vomiting by the simple solution of not eating, and avoiding passing out from pain by taking massive doses of pain-killers.

Migraine is like the pain of childbirth in the head and the discomfort of food poisoning in the stomach – it's about as similar to a headache as a knife stabbing might be to a pin-prick! The last few years of weekly migraines had taken more out of me than I cared to admit, and I had got to the point where the migraine would set in by Monday or Tuesday evening, to leave me by Saturday or Sunday. An existence – survival, not living!

But I felt relief. Now at last I could own up to feeling burnt-out, too exhausted to continue.

Chapter 2

The first signs

I sipped my wine, savouring the flavour of the crisp dry white, my usual order, as well as the warmth and bustle around me. The restaurant was packed, as it usually was on Friday nights – each table of diners was noisily enjoying food and company, waiters were rushing by, laden with plates of steaming food – and the smells of delicious Italian food were tantalising.

After we had said grace, my friend Leanne offered me the plate of crunchy, buttery herb and garlic bread, and we sat quietly for a few moments, as the week's tension and busyness ebbed away. We came here almost every Friday, hurrying up the street from her house, to the welcome we knew awaited us.

It was mid-winter (August) 1994, and for a couple of years we had been sharing our Friday evenings, mostly over wine and pasta at her local Italian restaurant. We talked about some of our week's events, laughing and sympathising, offering advice, consoling, and then reflecting on a whole stream of experiences that had flowed through our lives over the past year or so.

I forked up my last heap of pasta, and said: 'You know, I seem to be living on a giant roller-coaster – "God's roller-coaster". Every time life seems to settle down, off I go on some other hair-raising loop or dip. It's been like a switchback ride this past year for me!'

Leanne agreed, 'My life is a bit like that, too, and somehow our faith keeps us going, no matter what.'

'Yes, it's a bit like the wheels of the roller-coaster cart, keeping us clinging onto the rails somehow.'

I drained my glass, leant back, and thought about my experiences in 1993 and 1994. 'I think I've been on a fast and furious section of this particular roller-coaster for the last two years!'

If stress can begin to show up the symptoms of Alzheimer's, then 1993 and 1994 could have easily done it for me.

Life at work up to late 1992 had been stressful – but I still loved it, thriving on challenge. I headed up a division in the Prime Minister's department, of about 20–30 people. We advised the Prime Minister and his science minister on science and technology issues, we supported the chief scientist and his work, we managed the Cooperative Research Centre funding budget of around $130 million per year, and we were responsible for bringing to the government's attention important science and technology issues for the country's future.

We had also coped in 1992 with a change of Prime Minister, from Bob Hawke to Paul Keating. This was followed by changes of the science minister and his staff, as old allegiances were punished and rewarded; then of our departmental head, making way for new blood; and of the chief scientist, as ill health and all the changes took their toll.

It had been a tumultuous year – of changes, of uncertainty – but also of some successes and achievements. Science now received more attention in our department and in the Prime Minister's office, and we had managed to achieve some important gains for industrial research in particular. My working hours easily topped 70–80 hours a week, with a bulging briefcase coming home with me each night. But work was exciting and challenging, and I felt a bright future lay ahead in 1993–1994.

But I could not have been more wrong.

It was just a week or so before Christmas 1992. I had come home exhausted from a long day, and wondered when Ianthe would be home from her cricket camp – was it today or tomorrow? I sank into bed, she was still not home – maybe it must have been tomorrow she was meant to be back.

I woke up to a whispered 'Mum, could we talk? Now?' Ianthe was kneeling by my side of the bed. I blearily looked at the glowing red numerals on the clock – it was two or three in the morning. It must be serious I thought, and my heart started thumping.

We crept into her room, and sat on her bed. Ianthe said that her friend from cricket was still in the living room and had refused to go home until she told me what had happened on camp. Ianthe had been found, by this friend, unconscious, bleeding profusely from her slashed wrist. She had been taken to hospital, but was OK now. Our family doctor had been informed of this attempted suicide.

I was shocked, speechless, terribly sad, and just didn't know what to say or do. I sat there quietly gathering my thoughts, carefully thinking over each word I would say – this was a critical moment in my life – I must not get it wrong. I began to share a little of the despair that had haunted my days as a teenager, and in my twenties, without God and without hope. I, too, had felt that life was not worth living. Now I tried to comfort Ianthe and sent her friend home, thanking her for her help.

The next day, we talked some more, and agreed that she would go to talk to a counsellor. We also agreed we would not tell her dad, because we thought he would belittle her, and make cruel fun of her in some way.

The counsellor, after one session with her, asked me to come for counselling too. It was clear why, on my first visit. The attempt at suicide was a cry for help, a cry of desperation – on my behalf too – because Ianthe and I had been, and still were being, physically abused by my husband.

I went two or three times, more than Ianthe, but I, too, needed to talk, and to listen.

These sessions made me realise the harm my marriage was doing to my daughters. The fears were that they, too, might marry violent men; that they could suffer hidden emotional trauma for the rest of their lives; that Ianthe could not – would not – ever come home again while I stayed with my husband; and that I was actually scared of being killed one day. Could I – should I – live like this?

My choice had become very clear – the precious lives of Ianthe, Rhiannon and Micheline, or carry on pretending that my marriage was OK, when it wasn't.

Ironically, both Ianthe and I were hit during these few weeks of counselling. I felt devalued, emotionally fragile, and very shaky.

This precipitated my final decision to leave, and I started to look for a house to rent. I had another week or so of holiday left to deal with this. Some holiday!

I was sleepily drinking a morning cup of tea a week later, when the phone rang. It was for Ianthe. She said little, put the phone down and rushed to her room.

I followed her in and found her crying. Unprecedented! Only the previous week I had got a letter from the counsellor saying that one problem that had not really been resolved was that Ianthe felt somehow that it was wrong to cry. Maybe this was because she needed to feel strong, not powerless, in the face of violence.

The call was from the army. They had reviewed her files, and she was not medically fit, due to her poor eyesight, to be admitted to the Australian Defence Force Academy to study for her engineering degree. But she was due to start at the Academy in nine days' time! We had bought her things, and were packing up her room.

What about other university choices? The very next day was the last day to make second round choices for university places!

The army had tested her eyes back in October – so why did they suddenly discover this problem now! But arguments were not going to help, action was needed, so she and I took off for Sydney to apply in person to the clearing house for second round offers – it was too late for the mail.

It was a three-hour drive there and another three hours back. The summer heat was stifling – 40 degrees Celsius. Our eyes felt like fried eggs, our backs ran with sweat. Our emotions were a blank tangle of confusion, dismay, anger and frustration.

Over the next week or so we made the trip again, for medical reviews of the case, but the army would not be moved. There was no chance of organising a university place other than locally – there was no time to organise the upheaval of a move and so on. So she stayed in Canberra, and planned to do science/engineering at the Australian National University.

I went back to work in late January 1993, with my home life in turmoil. But at work, I was frenetically busy as usual. It retained a semblance of normality for me, even stability.

But then in March 1993, an election was called, and Keating – despite the pundits – won. 'A win for the true believers,' he called it. Yet again, it meant follow-on changes, even though the Prime Minister and his party retained government. Inevitably there were promotions, 'rewards', and reshuffles.

For my division, it meant a new science minister to work with. The previous minister had been a real sweetie, and was a delight to work with – polite, quiet, small stature and an alert and welcoming expression. He would ask questions, discuss issues, and always want to weigh up the pros and cons, and be willing to consider carefully any advice.

In the preparation for his Science Statement in mid-1992, I had often written up the minutes of a particular item from the Cabinet meeting, and then gone up to his office in the small hours, in the sure knowledge that he and his staff would be waiting to welcome me with a glass of white to sit back and review the success or otherwise of the proposals he had put to Cabinet.

We had worked well together, and shared a common hope of seeing science and technology gain more prominence on the national agenda. Tempered, of course, with the ever-present need to use any taxpayers' money wisely and frugally, and to encourage business investment wherever possible.

The new science minister was a tall bear of a man. He towered over me, and my eyes were level with about the bottom of his tie. He abounded in energy, in determination, and in forcefulness. He was in charge, and his views would prevail. He was determined to make changes to Australia's research institution, CSIRO – moving fisheries research out to form a new national marine institute, and moving the nuclear research body in to be managed by CSIRO. He was supported in these proposals by the chief scientist, who was a member of his office staff, although also working in our department supported by my division. A difficult situation, as it turned out.

I failed to see the logic in these proposals. It didn't seem to save money for the taxpayer, indeed it would cost money, nor did it seem to promise any extra benefit to the nation from research. This set the scene for an ongoing and tense confrontation.

Much of my time was spent in many telephone calls and meetings, briefing papers and, euphemistically speaking, 'full and frank' discussions with the minister and his staff! Frequently I'd be summoned to his office, shouted at, and I'd have to repeat – quietly but firmly – for the umpteenth time why I didn't think his plans were such a good idea.

People from the scientific and industrial community would ring me, complaining and giving their views and objections. The head of our department would call me into his office without notice to find out what on earth was happening. The Prime Minister's Office would summon me, wanting to know the latest in the stand-off.

And, of course, there were difficult silences and circular arguments with the chief scientist, who was normally a charming and welcoming family man, whose office in our department was just a corridor away from mine. Repeatedly I'd ask for a rationale to support the dramatic nature of all the changes proposed, but whatever was offered always fell far short of justifying what was needed.

In the end the proposals were dropped, but not before the science minister had rung my department complaining about me.

I peeked into Ianthe's room – her light was still on. It was the week after Easter and she was still struggling with glandular fever. But there she lay, with a huge book propped on her knees. I suggested she go to sleep. 'No, Mum, I've got exams and pracs all week – I *have* to study. But I don't know how I'll cope, I've got assignments due, too!'

Clearly the stress of doing a double science/engineering degree, with two faculties setting work independently of each other, made an almost impossible load. Together with her illness and the stress we were going through as a family, this was taking its toll.

'Why don't you just stop the course now?'

'But I'll fail if I stop now.'

'No, I mean withdraw, and take the rest of the year off.'

She was relieved, and amazed that I'd suggest that, but we agreed that next year she would try for Physiotherapy at Sydney University, with sports science at Canberra University as her second choice.

I said it would also be very helpful for me to have help at home while coping with the move to a new house – and it was indeed a real blessing to me for the rest of 1993, particularly the next few months.

It was a cold, bleakly grey Canberra autumn day, in May 1993, when I finally left my husband, taking with me 18-year-old Ianthe, 12-year-old Rhiannon and 8-year-old Micheline, as well as 16-year-old Buzz (our cat) and our recently acquired budgies.

We backed out of the driveway as the removal van was loading on our 'share' of the household goods. We had just experienced a weekend of trauma – arguments over each piece of cutlery, each item of furniture, each bed, each chair. I could have half, no more – so the girls could not even have each of their beds, nor their bed linen. I was wrung out and exhausted.

But our new home was a haven of peace. For the first time in my life, I looked forward to coming home from work. Each of us relished the chance to live together as a family, rather than be isolated in our rooms, avoiding the source of our fears.

No-one at work, apart from Margaret, my personal assistant, knew anything more than that I had moved house.

In the Budget of 1993 the division heads in my department had been asked to propose as many ways to save money as possible. I had put forward a number of minor savings proposals, but felt that everything in science had already been cut to the bone. There was nothing left to take.

But Cabinet decided otherwise. Instead of minor savings to the Australian Science and Technology Council, it was to have its budget slashed by 45 per cent, and its staff would be moved from independent offices immediately into my division.

For months I reeled with exhaustion, talking to staff, endlessly reviewing figures, and meeting with the Council members. There was a great deal of anger, resentment, mistrust – and much of this was directed at me. I was seen as the devil, complete with horns and a tail, who had caused this to occur.

No-one at work seemed to notice anything wrong with my performance. I coped, and coped well, succeeding in bringing about the changes the government wanted.

But at home, I let my guard down.

I was sitting at the kitchen table we had borrowed from Leanne, sipping my mug of tea before starting my busy round of Saturday morning activities – shopping, washing, cooking, cleaning… Ianthe was sitting up on the counter, talking to me, explaining, expounding. But she finally exploded in exasperation, 'Mum, I just can't believe you hold down such a responsible job. You're simply such an airhead at home!'

I mumbled about just feeling burnt-out and stressed. I needed 'brain time out' at home. 'You make the decision – I have to make too many of them at work.'

A few months later, Ianthe had just had a knee operation, so I was driving her to her regular tutoring session one evening. She directed me to the house, and I waited outside in the car with my 'in-tray'. I was never short of a huge pile of material to read, to comment on, and to make decisions upon.

Ianthe got back into the car. There was silence. 'Go on,' she said.

'Could you direct me?'

'But we only just came here! All right, just turn up here, left, up the hill.'

We reached the T-junction at the top. 'Well, you guess which way we go now!' she said jokingly, thinking anyone would know.

But I didn't, and guessed, and guessed wrong.

'I can't believe you just did that!' Ianthe said.

At work, I was suffering from thundering migraines. Each week they would set in by Monday afternoon/Tuesday morning, and only slowly lift at the weekend. Margaret would always know when I was sick – she'd see it in my eyes and say, 'You're looking a bit grey and pale. Are you OK? Shouldn't you go home? I could reorganise your schedule.'

But I always had far too many things to do, and would take handfuls of tablets to keep the pain and nausea under control, as well as reduce the migraine itself. I'd avoid eating in case I threw up, and would stand up slowly to avoid passing out from both the pain and all the tablets.

I sought permission from my departmental head to take extended leave from mid-November through to early February. He knew I had just had a gruesome year at work – with the CSIRO proposals and the new minister, and delivering a massive budget cut to an understandably unwilling and uncooperative body – and agreed. I think he also had an inkling that all was not well at home.

I rang my mum and dad, and said I was planning to visit, with Rhiannon and Micheline, and could they possibly lend me the money until the property settlement came through. They were thrilled, but refused to lend the money – instead they insisted on giving it to me. This was actually a great relief, as financially I was really struggling. I was paying rent for our home, as well as the full mortgage payments on the family home where my husband was staying, meeting lawyers' bills for the property settlement, and paying all the usual bills, school fees and so on.

Rhiannon, Micheline and I boarded the jumbo at Sydney, and I sank back in my seat, sipping orange juice and delighting in the excitement and apprehension I saw in my girls as they experienced the thrill of this huge machine powering up for take-off.

Ianthe had waved us off at the airport, after teary farewells. She had been selected to play national representative cricket, and was to play in Perth – a once-in-a-lifetime opportunity for her.

The girls and I did all the tourist things in London, and came home each evening to my parents' welcoming and cosy house, to inviting meals and to soft warm beds. We each (even me!) got pocket money from my dad – he clearly delighted in treating us, and we were overwhelmed by his generosity. We then visited my aunt and grandma in Belgium, and then spent some time seeing a few sights in Belgium, Holland, Germany and France – with me driving a car on the 'wrong' (or right) side of the road. I managed – but only just!

It was freezing cold in the northern hemisphere January. Even Eurodisney was deserted – but the girls got to go fourteen times on the roller-coaster with no waits between! We made the most of our time, seeing castles, flooded rivers, and the changing cultural scenery of a land that has so much history.

We then started to turn back for Australia and the warmth. We stopped at Hong Kong to visit my sister, Denny, and her family, spending a few weeks thawing out, and having some family time together.

I sank back into Denny's leather couch at one stage and said: 'I still feel burnt-out and exhausted!'

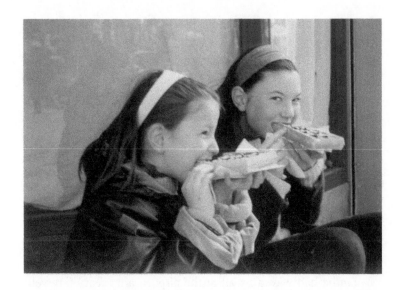

Overseas trip in 1993; Micheline and Rhiannon in Brussels eating waffles

She took me for a new hairdo, a new outfit. I was much spruced up on the outside, but just as ragged and exhausted on the inside.

A nut-brown Ianthe met us at the airport, delighted to welcome us home in early February 1994. She was a little fragile, as my husband had been ringing her at all hours, embarking on some very strange conversations. So much so, that she had gone to stay with Leanne.

I'd only been back a few days when my husband started to come round, often very late at night, quite distraught, to talk.

The stress of my leaving him, and then going overseas for such a long period, clearly had been the trigger to a major breakdown. Also, the property settlement had just gone through, and even though he would get more than 60 per cent, the reality had hit home – he would now have to vacate the family home, sell up, and make moves to finding some way to support himself. But he was in no mental state to cope rationally with any of this.

The February summer nights were warm and balmy, so I would lock the security door, and if and when he arrived, we would hold tense and very weird conversations through the wire mesh about things he accused me or others of doing, or things he believed he had done. Many times I would say, 'These incidents, I know, are very real for you, but I really don't remember them – they really didn't – couldn't have happened.'

I felt inadequate to deal with these problems.

It became quite serious after a week or so, so I rang Margaret and asked her to reorganise some meetings so that I could take much of the day off work in order to seek medical help for him.

Later in the day I went back to work, as if nothing had happened. 'A bit of a medical crisis at home,' I said.

Only a month or so later, the government decided to reshuffle ministerial responsibilities, and there would be a new science minister. Hooray! I thought – anything has got to be better than my ongoing difficulties with the current one.

But the government also decided that the current science minister would gain responsibility for the Cooperative Research Centres Program, and that its staff were to be moved from my division in the Prime Minister's Department, to his department. Maybe this was some kind of trade-off.

For me, it was a traumatic time. We were informed in the morning, and by that afternoon the staff would no longer be in my division. Also, the painstaking work we had just done to accommodate the extra Australian Science and Technology Council staff had been pointless, as there would now be plenty of room!

The office was in turmoil, staff were unhappy, confusion reigned.

Yet again, I felt as if I was rushing down another loop on my switchback roller-coaster.

I was still getting debilitating migraines, more and more frequently. I thought maybe what I needed was a change at work. So I went for a couple of interviews – and unlike any of my previous efforts to get a new job, I was unsuccessful each time. The interviews were, for me, a source of panic as I kept 'losing the plot' in mid-sentence, or failing to grasp the essence of a question and answering capably.

My lack of success had Ianthe really worried. I had never failed to get a job I sought before, and she began to worry about whether – in her language – I was 'losing it'.

Well, as far as I was concerned everything was OK, but I was very stressed and all these problems were only too easy to write off as due to work pressures, combined with the difficulties I was going through at home.

Each night I'd stagger home after collecting Micheline from after-school care, with my in-tray under one arm, and a bulging briefcase dangling at the end of the other. I'd be greeted with: 'What's for dinner, Mum?' The cupboards were often empty, and my energy for cooking non-existent. Cheese toast was often the answer!

Looking back now, I can see that one early sign of the onset of Alzheimer's may well have been when I went for new glasses in July 1994.

The optometrist placed the awkward heavy metal frame on my nose and then started to slide round the lenses, each time asking what I could see. Each time, my answer was the same, 'Nothing yet. We'll have to wait until the fog clears.'

He was puzzled as to why my eyes took so long to adjust to each new lens.

But now I think that my reaction times were already slowing down, back then.

Two incidents in mid-1994 really shook me up, as they occurred in the true centre of my life – my girls.

Micheline had been complaining of a sore hip for a week or so, and finally I got her to a doctor one Saturday morning, in between the shopping, cleaning, washing and so on. He referred her for ultrasound on the Monday. The grainy, shifting, black and white picture showed a caterpillar-like angry-looking appendix. I whisked her to the specialist and she was in hospital the next day. That week I was an automaton – at home making lunches, cooking, tidying up, at the computer till the small hours – at the hospital, sitting by her bed before work, at lunch and after work, clacking away on my laptop – at work, chairing meetings, writing, making calls, negotiating. Bleary-eyed with exhaustion, I was delighted when her bite into a cheeseburger by the Friday signalled to the specialist that she was finally well enough to come home!

Life returned to normal – for a while.

Rhiannon had been given some money by her grandparents to buy a horse. She was looking at a few, and trying them out.

One bright Saturday morning I drove her to a paddock about half an hour away, where this stringy-looking grey Arab rolled its bloodshot eyes at us. After some pre-sales pitch about how wonderful he was, Rhiannon got on for a ride.

He was off, falling over his own legs like a clumsy, gangly schoolboy, but each time Rhiannon held on. Then he gathered speed, racing round and round the paddock, like a slingshot gaining speed to spin out to freedom beyond the fence. Rhiannon realised what the horse had in mind, and had the good sense to throw herself off before things got too much out of control.

I saw her in slow motion, sailing high up in the air like a puppet free of its strings, her arms and legs flailing. She hit the ground like a rag doll, bounced, bounced again with her head wobbling to and fro, and then crumpled into a heap. It took what felt like hours to reach her, lying there deathly still, her nose and mouth buried in the soft earth. I touched her, spoke to her, praying under my breath. After what seemed an age, she stirred, mumbled, spat out earth, and rolled onto her back. Slowly we got her up, and the rest of the day was spent in hospital, as she was monitored for concussion. Miraculously, she was unharmed.

In September 1994, I was presented with the Public Service Medal, for services to science and technology – but felt embarrassed and inadequate for such an honour. I had received this award in the Queen's Birthday Honours List in June, but life had been so stressful, so busy, that it was hard to focus on what this meant.

I remember rushing back to Canberra from a meeting in Melbourne, with a thundering migraine, to participate in the medal-awarding ceremony at the Governor-General's house. It all seemed like a dream through a haze of pain. I rushed back to Melbourne that evening, as I had to chair an important meeting the very next day.

Little wonder I was suffering the symptoms of stress, or at least thought all my symptoms were from stress alone!

I took an hour off work later that same month, to pop down to the Family Court, to the hearing of the divorce case. It only took ten minutes, but it lifted a twenty-year burden from my shoulders.

The following month I finally received the money from the property settlement, and could at last pay all my debts – and think about looking for a small house to buy for me and the girls. At long last we could also stop worrying if there was enough money for the housekeeping!

At the end of 1994 I took a three-week break over Christmas. Things had settled down at work, and home life was peaceful and uneventful. As usual, I 'went on holiday' to my favourite location – home! To be a mum to my three daughters, and to potter around with them and go places with them in their holidays.

I really felt free of stress at last. We had just heard that Ianthe had finally got in to do Physiotherapy at Sydney University, after a year of sports science at Canberra University, and everything seemed to be falling into place. My ex-husband seemed to be quite stable, the girls were happy at school and at home. I felt everything at work was in good order, and I had exciting ideas for new directions for our division. I felt able to cope easily, and wanted to enjoy life.

I spent my holiday buying terracotta pots for our rented house, and choosing plants. What a delight it was to run my fingers through the soil, looking carefully at each plant, and watering, feeding and generally taking the time to 'watch the plants grow'.

But when I had five migraines in that short but restful holiday break, it was the last straw. I had to get rid of these migraines somehow. I changed my family doctor and my new one was sympathetic, having been a migraine sufferer herself.

I'd already tried most migraine cures – changing my diet, vitamins and so on. Also people kept sending me articles on all sorts of treatments.

The new doctor was methodical in her approach, asking me to keep a headache diary, and then trying most combinations of tablets – both old and new migraine treatments – and still I got weekly migraine attacks. By Tuesday I'd be well into it, and only get well by Sunday, ready for another week at work. And now I was getting so sick that I had to go home more and more often – something I had never done before.

By early March 1995, I was feeling more and more stressed and confused.

Rhiannon, Micheline and I would pile into the car each morning, in a great rush. Lunches had been hastily made, bags packed and my briefcase and in-tray thrown into the back of the car. Turn left out of the driveway, right at the end of my street, and down to the T-junction. But which one was this? I had two T-junctions to negotiate. 'Do I turn left or right here?'

Rhiannon and Micheline could not believe what they were hearing. 'We always turn right here!' they chorused, with some amusement.

No-one knew at work that often I got lost on the way there – neither did my doctor. It was just stress, as far as I was concerned. I had too much on my mind, that's all.

In early April 1995, my doctor decided to send me for routine brain CT (computerised tomography). I fitted in these scans on a frenetic Thursday, between two stressful meetings. It was actually quite a treat to lie quietly for ten minutes while being scanned! The CT was basically a total and detailed picture of my brain, built up from many X-rays, each of a thin slice (pictorially, not literally!) through the brain. The doctor wanted to make sure there was no physical cause – no tumours or anything like that – for my migraines.

I went back to the doctor on the 10th of April. She took out the scans from their large envelope, looked at them and the radiologist report carefully, and said that although there were no tumours, there was quite a surprise in that there appeared to be generalised atrophy (wasting away) of the brain. She insisted I go to see a specialist neurologist that very afternoon and arranged an appointment with the nearest and most readily available one in Canberra.

The specialist looked at the scans, checked my reflexes and general neurological status. Then he asked me about any other symptoms. I related how I was really quite stressed out and felt burnt-out and exhausted. He was the first outside my family to hear that I had sometimes taken the wrong turning on my usual route to work, that I occasionally 'blanked out' in mid-sentence, and I couldn't remember people's names – even those of my staff at work. To me these all seemed simply to be symptoms of stress, and what I felt I needed was a long restful break and then everything would be all right.

The specialist said very little, but referred me for more scans – this time MRI (magnetic resonance imaging).

Now I was getting concerned – maybe this was more than just stress. Even I could tell there was a big hole in the middle of my brain, and lots of space around it. The CT scan of my head looked like a black and white picture of a shrivelled walnut!

That very night, I had a large formal function to attend at Parliament House, the award of the Australia Prize for science and technology. I would have a chance to meet up with colleagues from around Australia, catch up on news, swap ideas, and rekindle my excitement for a technological future. But my head was pounding and my mind was in turmoil. I went through the motions of circulating, talking to people, greeting former colleagues. It was all like a bad dream.

The migraine pursued me home, beleaguered me all night, and totally debilitated me the next day. It was the worst I had experienced in a long time, and I excused myself from a meeting that next morning, and went home to bed.

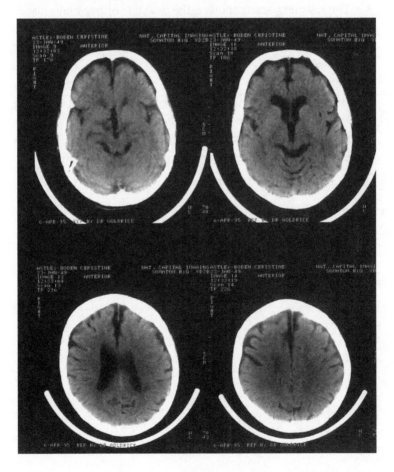

Computerised Tomography (CT) scans taken in April 1995

A few weeks later, on the 4th of May 1995, I had the MRI scan. This was an even more detailed picture of my brain, made by sensing the vibration-like response of all my minute brain atoms to a large electromagnet pulsing around my head. Totally painless but a bit claustrophobic – lying on a metal table and being slid into a very small, narrow tunnel around which the magnet made very noisy grinding sounds, clunks and clicks. And staying there for what seemed like hours, but in reality was probably only 15–20 minutes.

The resulting scans showed the 'walnut' of my brain just as shrivelled as ever, so I thought up all sorts of excuses as to why I couldn't get back to the specialist with my scans for another week or so.

And of course you know the rest of the story, as far as that fateful visit to the first, Canberra-based specialist went, shocking me with the first diagnosis of Alzheimer's disease.

And, yes, I was still convinced I was far too young, and that something else had to explain why my brain was wasting away.

Chapter 3

The second opinion

'My wife's a physio,' the specialist said, having asked Ianthe what she was studying in Sydney. 'What year are you in?' Ianthe explained that she was in first year, but had just completed a year of sports science.

It was the 30th of May, just eight days after the first diagnosis, and we were in the second specialist's office. This new specialist was clearly going to treat us very much as people, not just as medical cases, and to explain as much as possible at each step of the tests.

These tests were extensive. The first step took two days, and began with a complete gamut of blood tests, to rule out any infections that could have caused the damage to my brain, including AIDS, which can cause dementia. The blood tests also looked for hormone deficiencies, or the presence of any toxic substances. These can also cause dementia, and if corrected can be cured. Unfortunately nothing showed up.

I also had a SPECT (single photon emission computed tomography) scan. This was a bit like MRI, in that it relied on detecting changes in atoms around my brain, and like the X-ray CT in that it built up a detailed picture from a whole series of tiny 'slices' through my brain. But unlike both of these, which looked at structural changes in the brain, the SPECT would look at how my brain was actually functioning, specifically how it was using oxygen.

I was injected with a low-level radioactive substance, as a sort of label in my blood that could be seen by the scanner as the blood flowed around my brain. An hour or so after the injection, my brain was scanned to see whether the flow of blood was abnormal. And yes, unfortunately it was. Not only was there very little activity where my brain had wasted away, but also other areas showed reduced blood flow.

It confirmed functionally what had been seen physically on the other scans – where there was less brain, there was less function. And, even worse, areas of brain that appeared normal on the other scans were not functioning normally.

On the 14th and 15th of August 1995, I went to see a clinical psychologist (one that diagnoses any diseases, rather than talks to you about psychological problems) to have psychometric tests. The tests took a total of four hours over two days, and I found them exhausting, going home to sleep each day.

But they weren't complicated tests – they only consisted of some very simple tasks such as trying to memorise a few shopping lists, putting cartoon pictures in the right order to tell a story, repeating strings of six or seven numbers, forwards and backwards. It was peculiar that I found it easier to repeat them backwards because the last few numbers were still resonating inside my brain.

The final tests, finding my way through an electronic maze, defeated me! No matter how many times I tried, I simply couldn't remember which route to take. No wonder I had taken a wrong turning or two on the way to work!

These tests showed that I had a very good capacity to perform tasks that I had learned in earlier years – like remembering the meanings of words, and such things as knives belong to forks, salt to pepper and so on. But when it came to learning anything new, my performance fell to abysmal levels. Again the tests were consistent with a diagnosis of Alzheimer's disease. Things weren't looking too good!

The specialist asked if I would be prepared to go overnight into hospital on the 21st of August, to have a lumbar puncture and a small bowel biopsy, as well as have a final scan. I agreed, of course, as I was only too keen to find some other cause for my brain damage and reduced functioning.

But what, I asked, does my bowel have to do with my brain? He explained that a rare disease of the bowel, called Whipple's disease, could cause brain damage like mine, and could be cured with antibiotics over the course of a year. Hooray, I thought, I can be cured! (Even my rector, Chris, at church, when asking everyone to pray for me over the few weeks of these final tests, said he wondered if God would mind if we prayed that I had a specific disease, rather than the usual praying for healing.)

The lumbar puncture would show up any infections that I may have had, even in the past, that could explain the damage to my brain.

The scan was the final step in all my tests. It would look at how my brain was using glucose in my blood, and whether its functioning was impaired in the typical pattern expected for Alzheimer's. This test was PET (positron emission tomography) scanning. Yet again a picture of my brain's function was to be built up from many thin image 'slices', and also again a 'label' of slightly radioactive glucose would be injected into me, and my brain scanned to see where this label went and how it was used.

There are only two PET scanners in Australia, both at universities and both used mainly for research. I was tested by the research team at the University of Sydney. It took all afternoon for the tests, and before starting the procedures were carefully explained to me. First my arms were to be put in huge rubber gloves that were inserted into a warm water bath, whilst I was blindfolded and lay quietly for an hour or so. Then I would have needles inserted into both arms: one to feed in the radioactive glucose label, the other to take out samples of my blood to test for this glucose. I would then be wheeled into a scanning tunnel – yet again, I thought – and strapped to the table with a mask fitted to my face and preventing any slight movement whilst the scanner was scanning.

I lay in a darkened room, with ear plugs and a blindfold and a Hannibal Lecter-type mask strapping my head down to a long cold steel table. The scanner clicked and clunked around my head. The research team, who used this as a research tool as well as a diagnostic tool, sat outside – twiddling knobs and taking notes, whilst I offered up my brain metabolism for their scrutiny.

I had been lying there – isolated from busy Sydney clattering on the outside – for about an hour when at last, after what seemed to be all afternoon, I was helped out of all this paraphernalia. And there, sitting quietly by my side, was my best friend Karen from Sydney, who had taken time out from her research to sit beside me during the test, without me knowing, and to pray as I underwent this discomfort.

She had a remarkable experience while praying. She was quite willing to sit there and pray all the time, but had felt she was being reassured that I was safe in God's grace and there was no need to ask for anything. This was a comfort and reassurance to both of us, giving us the peace we had sought.

It had been a long afternoon of lying flat on my back on a trolley or a scanning table, with blindfold and mask on. I was very confused and disoriented when I finally had to make my way out into the world again and, thank God, Karen was there to help me!

The research team talked to my specialist the very next day, and confirmed that the impaired way my brain was functioning clearly pointed to a diagnosis of Alzheimer's disease. A while later, the specialist also got the lumbar puncture and bowel biopsy results – both negative. I had no infection or disease that could explain my brain damage. Basically, he had now ruled out any other known cause for the physical deterioration in my brain and the decline in my brain function, apart from Alzheimer's.

There is no test that can definitely confirm this diagnosis – except a biopsy of my brain. Given that there is already less of my brain than there ought to be, they will wait until I am dead before cutting up my brain and saying whether I had Alzheimer's or not!

On the 15th of September 1995, the specialist formally recommended that I seek immediate retirement from work. He prescribed tacrine for me, which acts by raising the levels of a neurotransmitter (or natural chemical messenger in the brain). This helps the remaining parts of my brain work to the best of their ability, and keeps me functioning well for as long as possible.

It was not a cure, he said, and in about a third of patients it had no effect, in another third it slowed the decline in function, and in the last third it could even give some improvement. But it would take at least six months to find out in what third I would be.

That six months was difficult.

I had already gone through a terrible four months of fear, of uncertainty, between the first and the second diagnosis. I had tried to read about the disease, but wanted desperately to keep hoping it was not Alzheimer's, so only cursorily glanced at a lot of the material. It was all so depressing – no cure, no treatment, no hope. And even the one Christian book I had glanced through gave me little courage – except the hope of heaven.

But now I needed to become more positive, to face up to the reality of what lay ahead for us as a family. I drew mostly on my faith, with a strong dose of humour, and seasoned this with my natural tendency to want to take on new challenges. I began to adjust to the diagnosis, to accept the dramatic change in my life, and to study as much as I could about Alzheimer's. I learned a great deal that I did not know, and have written some of this down to share with others (in Appendix I).

I think the worst part of the six months was just not knowing how fast I would deteriorate. I read all the available books by other Alzheimer's sufferers – but they never had quite the same problems as each other, or as me. It's not like other diseases, where there is a standard set of symptoms. At least in the early stages it seems to be as individual as the patients themselves, whose very personality and individuality is being eroded.

Each patient declines in his or her very own way, losing different abilities at different times. So would I be able to write next week? Would I be able to calculate my finances on next month's bank statement? Would I get lost after taking the girls to school tomorrow? What will it be like to be demented? How are my girls going to cope with my terrible deterioration, and eventual death maybe in 6–8 years' time? All these questions, and more, kept running through my mind, and I had to work through a lot of fear and anxiety.

But 'popular' misunderstandings about Alzheimer's disease didn't help me and my girls much – we were up against more than just the disease itself.

Who will I be when I die?

Chapter 4

At least you can't die from it! – wrong!

'What's the hurry? She's hardly at death's door!' said the person dealing with my case for retirement on medical grounds, to the personnel people at my work.

This was not an uncommon reaction. Even friends and family said at first, 'At least you can't die from Alzheimer's! You'll just be a little more forgetful.' These misconceptions, about a disease which is the fourth most common cause of death in Australia, dogged us as a family from the time of the first diagnosis.

After the final diagnosis by the second specialist in mid-September 1995, I faced the task of seeking retirement on medical grounds, before I got too sick to cope with the whole process. And no-one could even tell me how long I would be able to sign my name, let alone go through the tortuous process of applying to my superannuation company for a pension.

My battles with this superannuation company, when trying to follow the specialist's advice to seek retirement from work, epitomise the misunderstandings about Alzheimer's as a killer disease. The company's board arranged for me to be examined by its own doctor in October 1995. This doctor agreed with the diagnoses of the first and second specialists, and their opinions that I should cease work immediately. He recommended that I be medically retired from work as soon as possible.

The company's board then asked a panel in Sydney to provide an assessment of my case. I and the personnel people at my work were confident that retirement would then follow relatively easily. But this was not to be!

The Assessment Panel – a firm called something like Bloggs, Bloggs and Bloggs (the board refused to give us the actual name, unless I applied formally and paid a standard fee) – recommended in November 1995 that I return to work to be retrained in a lower level job!

I was overcome with anxiety as I read these words – how could I go back, when even life at home was so difficult! Each day was a battle to remember how to do things, to approach each task slowly enough so I had time to work through my thoughts, and to keep in mind what I was meant to be doing at any one time and where everyone else was and why. And almost each week I'd reach the point of exhaustion from some simple series of events that took me beyond my now very constrained abilities.

Presumably the superannuation company thought I was pretending to be a bit brainless so that I could stop work! Over the sixteen years I had contributed to my superannuation fund, I had accumulated the nine months of sick leave I was still using – hardly the sign of a malingerer!

The suggestion that I return to work for retraining appalled all the medical people associated with my case, as well as my department and my friend Jeffi, the librarian at the Alzheimer's Association. We all knew at least the basics of Alzheimer's: that the first capacity lost is holding a job, and that, in particular, learning any new tasks is almost impossible for someone with the disease. And here the suggestion was that I should not only continue to try to hold a job, but learn a completely new one, with a whole range of new tasks, new places to find, new colleagues to recognise!

It was a devastating time for us as a family. I was very worried about how I could possibly cope. It would mean driving in heavy traffic, shopping in busy, noisy shopping centres, remembering a whole list of home and work issues, learning (or rather coping with the embarrassment of never remembering) so many new things. I became very distressed thinking how this would affect us as a family, and how it would be likely to make me very sick, with continual migraines again, and rapidly increasing confusion as stress began to take its toll on my diseased brain. The specialist had warned that stress would exacerbate the progress of the disease.

Ianthe decided to take a year off university, as there seemed to be no other option for us – there was simply no way I would be able to cope without a great deal of help with home life, nursing and assistance when sick, and guidance in making the decisions and choices of a working mother. As I no longer had any room for her at home, since we had moved to the townhouse when she left for university, she and her friend, Rachel, managed to find a small flat nearby, just a few minutes' walk from my back gate. She tried a variety of casual jobs to pay rent and living costs, and eventually found herself a part-time job.

My specialist recommended I seek legal advice, but fortunately the sympathetic and efficient personnel people from my department reassured me and said they would fight this on my behalf. They talked with my specialist, who arranged for some follow-up psychometric tests in January 1996, and these confirmed my steady deterioration.

They arranged for my specialist to write another letter in February 1996 which laid it on the line – that I would need help with personal care in about a year or so, and would need full nursing care in a few years. He said it would be 'extreme cruelty' to attempt to retrain me at a new workplace. He also noted that life expectancy was usually about 6–8 years from diagnosis, and that given the exhaustive nature of the tests (physical tests, including magnetic resonance, positron emission tomography, radioactive tracers, and lumbar puncture; as well as psychological tests), it would be pointless challenging the final diagnosis.

The 7th of March 1996 was a sunny cloudless morning. I was tidying up the kitchen after the girls had gone to school, when the phone rang. It was the personnel manager from my department. The board had just agreed to retire me, and a letter was on its way. He assured me that I need not worry any more, and that he and his staff would help in all the administrative steps to be taken.

I was speechless with relief, mumbling some words of thanks. After gathering my breath again, I phoned Ianthe at work, stumbling over the words but somehow managing to get the message across!

She and her friend, Rachel, arrived that evening with champagne, soft drinks and chocolates. We all sat on our balcony in the warm autumn dusk, overwhelmed with relief and joy. Ianthe managed to hit a nearby house roof with the champagne cork, and amidst bubbles and cheers we settled down to making plans for our immediate future.

It was too late for Ianthe to go back to university, but we decided to make the most of our year together, whilst I was still relatively well, and able to cope with a quiet and simple life as a single mum.

But our traumatic experience with the superannuation company shows how statistics can mask personal reality:

- statistically, most Alzheimer's patients are older, and by some quirk of this brain disease, seem to last longer than younger patients – having life expectancies of 15–20 years.

- but 2 per cent of Alzheimer's sufferers are under the age of sixty-five and, unlike older patients, may have a much shorter life expectancy (as short as 5–10 years), possibly because of a faster progression of the disease.

So therefore actuarial data (no doubt used by my superannuation company) might well point to people being healthy for many years – or dying of something other than Alzheimer's in older patients – because 98 per cent of Alzheimer's patients are a lot older, and can last some fifteen years. They may indeed die of something else first.

And statistics are a very poor indicator of something as little understood as Alzheimer's. Often life expectancies relate more to the quality of care offered, as well as other genetic or external risk factors.

Chapter 5

You look so well! – if only I had cancer!

I sat with a couple of friends in my garden, sharing a pot of tea and some biscuits.

'You look so well!' one friend said.

'Yes,' said the other, 'I don't think I've ever seen you looking so well.'

But how did they expect me to look? How are you meant to look to the outside world when you have Alzheimer's disease?

For younger sufferers, we don't *look* to you as if we have Alzheimer's – you know, white-haired, doddery, frail. We don't look that old, we are often fit in our physical bodies, and so you don't know anything is wrong with us.

The time I now have at home, to rest, to eat, to garden, means that I look better than I have ever done before. I'm now quite normal in build rather than thin, and no longer appear pale, drawn and ill, as I was at work with continual migraines.

Unfortunately I have a disease of the brain, so you just can't see the diseased bit of me. My outer shell is fine, it's just my mental powerhouse that is on the blink! What's wrong with me is inside my head. I'll probably look well until shortly before I die, when my brain finally forgets how to run my body. Unlike other diseases, such as cancer, people who don't know I am dying will see me as a perfectly fit person who just behaves a bit oddly.

In early 1997 I had an unusual spot appear and grow larger on my leg. I joked – but more than half seriously – 'Maybe it's cancer, and if I do not get it treated, I could die as "me", not some very altered person who is totally confused and not connecting with life around her!' It turned out to be a wart. Although it was large and malicious-looking, it was totally harmless. I was actually disappointed that it was not cancer, as I still sought some release from a death of my mind by slow degrees.

If I were to die of cancer, I would still be the real me, the one I know, the one my family and friends know – mother of my three girls and member of my church 'family'. When I die of Alzheimer's, who will I be when I die? Even though friends and family repeatedly reassure me that I will always retain the essential 'me' right to the end, only my head knows this, but my heart still does not accept it.

Alzheimer's disease is a terrible thing for us as a family to face up to – that slowly there might be less and less of 'the old me', as my brain slowly erodes away. The brain is, in a way, what defines us, gives us our sense of consciousness, of being in a world and able to interact with that world. It, too, I feel, is what gives us the ability to pray, to communicate with God.

I am scared of the prospect of eventually not recognising my surroundings and not knowing who my girls are, or being able to greet my friends. Surely that will be a lonely and frightening place to be – always somewhere unfamiliar, surrounded by strangers, and nothing you recognise to turn to. Will I still be able to hold onto my faith in God?

At least with cancer there is a chance, however small, of full recovery. Who has ever heard of someone getting better from properly diagnosed Alzheimer's? In the past all sorts of dementias (caused by depression, hormone deficiency or toxic substances) were all lumped together and called Alzheimer's. But many of those other causes of dementia can be cured. And that is why I had so many tests, to rule out all possible curable forms of dementia, and to find a cause for the brain damage that was so clearly visible on X-ray, let alone on the other more specialised forms of brain scan.

So Alzheimer's expected to be is a one-way street; true, it's relatively slow, but it is inexorable. Death by small steps. Friends and relatives lose you by minute amounts each day, each week, each month, each year. So perhaps they will get used to this slowly evolving new person, until they have forgotten what you were really like before your brain started disappearing. That's why I'm glad we have bought a video camera. At least there will be some record of who I was when I was more or less really me, and not the diseased me.

And my very dear friend, Karen, has said she will always remember me at the various stages. She has travelled this road with her father. I trust her to be there for me until the end.

My daughters, too, will always remember, I know, but for them there will be so much pain and grief that this will be the hardest part for them – watching me disappear by small steps, becoming someone different each day.

The material I have read talks of being 'stripped to the core' with Alzheimer's, and so although the outer layers are gone, the essence of what makes the person an individual remains, and this includes their spirituality. Maybe this should reassure me.

Oliver Sacks said, in a recent *7.30 Report* interview, that Alzheimer's sufferers don't lose their essential selves. True, maybe, but I know that I have changed a lot already. I am more stretched out somehow, more linear, more step by step in my thoughts. I have lost that vibrancy, the buzz of interconnectedness, the excitement and focus I once had. I have lost the passion, the drive that once characterised me. I'm like a slow motion version of my old self – not physically, but mentally. It's not all bad, as I have more inner space in this linear mode to listen, to see, to appreciate clouds, leaves, flowers... I am less driven and less impatient. And Karen certainly prefers me this way!

But am I really still me?

We are each a kaleidoscope of personality, which makes up every facet of who we are. But often we are limited in our range of expression of this multi-faceted person, because of our busyness, the demands and constraints, the expectations of our lives. I believe that God knows us in our entirety, each and every part of this kaleidoscope of who we are. As I unfold before God, as this disease unwraps me, opens up the treasures of what lies within my multifold personality, I can feel safe as each layer is gently opened out.

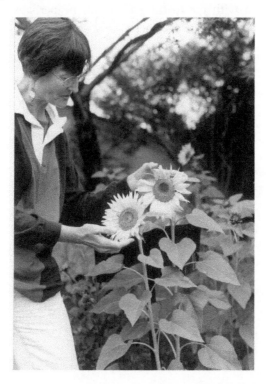

Christine admiring her sunflowers in 1995; watching flowers grow – her new passion – in her slow-motion version of herself

The fullness of who I once was will be seen in the simplicity of who I am within, surrounded by layer upon layer of memories. These memories form the kaleidoscopic perspectives of all the many expressions of my being over my lifetime: as a child, daughter, granddaughter and sister, as a student and young adult, as a wife and mother, as a friend, as a researcher, an editor, an information officer, policy manager and senior public servant, as a member of St George's church and a Cursillo team member, and as a writer of this book.

In each of these aspects of my life, the centre of my being was always there within, expressing itself in these many forms of me. This unique essence of 'me' is at my core, and this is what will remain with me to the end. I will be perhaps even more truly 'me' than I have ever been.

Chapter 6

A terminal illness – so why are we ashamed of it?

Alzheimer's is not a mental illness – I don't need a shrink. It is an organic disease of the brain, that eventually leads to death. I have outlined in Appendix I as best I can what I have gleaned from my investigations (personally motivated) over the year or so since being diagnosed with this disease.

Basically some cells of the brain become diseased and tangled, confused and no longer able to function. The cells affected are those making up our personality, our behaviour, our thinking, our memory. These cells are mainly at the front of the brain, around the temples and behind the eyes.

The disease has little effect on body movement and function, which are actually controlled by a relatively small area of the brain. The largest effect is on the 'higher order' brain cells – those that make us who we are. Eventually, so much is destroyed that the brain can no longer run the body (you forget, for example, how to swallow), and you fall into a coma and die. So people can't actually see much happening. We don't shake, we can walk…but our behaviour begins to change.

In its early stages it creeps up on you, subtly altering your behaviour and how you cope with life. Everything becomes more stressful, and that stress in itself can exacerbate the disease. In my case, I was lucky to be diagnosed in the early stages.

But what of a person who lives alone, and is already retired? They may have family who rarely visit, and have no work colleagues. They may indeed have no club or church, no-one who knows them and their circumstances. Say an elderly widow(er) gets the first signs. Who will notice?

It is unlikely in those mild to moderate stages of the disease that an Alzheimer's sufferer will keep up their social or even family contacts, because in the early stages we tend to avoid what are for us difficult situations. Conversations, chats, children playing, background music – all these are very hard for us to deal with because our brains work so much harder to sort out the competing sounds and sights in our surroundings so as to make sense of them.

And it is often not much better for those who have close family and friends, who know us well and watch us change. They become ashamed of our odd behaviour, and annoyed at our peculiarities and frustrated with our anti-social tendencies. Certainly at first they'd just get very irritated at our 'playing up'. Why can't we be nicer, more tolerant, more like we used to be? Why do we repeat ourselves, badger them for help, interrupt their conversations…?

Even once a diagnosis is made, families are still left to cope with very difficult behaviour, and are often ashamed, pretending nothing is wrong. We would not be ashamed of our relative or friend with cancer, heart attack or stroke, so why are we so ashamed of a disease that attacks us just as physically, but in the brain?

But it is far easier to say your beloved family member has cancer, than to say he or she has dementia – they are no longer 'normal', no longer as easily acceptable in social settings – no-one knows quite how to treat someone with dementia.

Is it because we don't look sick? Is it because we seem to behave as if we have a mental illness?

Should you talk to us as if we are 'normal'? Should you try to ignore us (not too obviously, of course)? Should you talk to our 'carer'?

But we can't help the way we are – we know there is something terribly wrong with us, and we seem to be losing touch with even who we are, all our feelings and our ability to express ourselves. We need all the help and support we can get. Don't hide us away – involve us, let us still experience the joy of living, with the help of your memory, your abilities, and your patience.

Perhaps we need to rethink our approach to this terminal illness, and not only continue to give plenty of support to the carers (who need compassion, counselling and lots of practical help), but also support the sufferers (who will lose their capacity to think, to function, to be themselves). They, too, need help to overcome the shame of the disease, to alleviate some of its effects with modern drugs, and to understand more about what is happening to them.

Indeed, carers do have a terrible time in the moderate to severe stages, and need all the support they can get – emotional, physical and spiritual. At these later stages, we sufferers, it is true, may need only appropriate physical care, and gentle understanding and management of our emotional and spiritual needs.

But in the early stages of the disease, we sufferers need your support, too. We have been given what, I think, is the worst diagnosis anyone can hear. You know there is no cure and no treatment, no hope, that you are going to lose everything that makes you who you are, and that you will die not knowing your family or your surroundings.

I have found that even the Alzheimer's Association tends to direct its attention mostly to carers. We sufferers seem to be ignored – on the assumption, perhaps, that we are 'too far gone' to care. But with more reliable and earlier diagnosis, as well as the availability of drugs to keep sufferers functioning better for longer in the early to moderate stages, we need to remember the sufferers too.

It is very scary to be diagnosed with an incurable dementing disease. Try to imagine it – you are faced with the knowledge that you are going to lose all your normal mental functions over a period of years, and no-one can tell you exactly what will happen when, nor how long it will take.

What's it like, having Alzheimer's?

Chapter 7

Clinging to a precipice with my fingernails

'That always happens to me!' my friend exclaimed, after I had just described a bit of difficulty I was having finding the right words, and participating in social conversations at our Bible study group. I smiled, and we carried on talking for a short while, but inside I was crying out 'Why can't she understand what it's really like!' But I knew that she was only somehow just trying to make me feel better, less of a freak, more 'normal'.

But I know exactly what it is like *not* to have Alzheimer's and to be normal – with a few small slip-ups every now and then, along the lines of 'that always happens to me'. Remember, I used to be free of this disease, too, once!

And I know only too well that this is *not* what it is like now – it's totally foggy in my head, and everything takes lots of effort and control. Without a huge effort, I make slip-ups all the time, but 'normal' people, don't need this amount of effort just to keep on track.

I'm OK as long as I am really trying hard, I am well rested and not at all tired. Then I could almost pass for normal. But inside me, it feels as if I am clinging to a precipice by my fingernails. It takes all my effort to stay where I am, and to lose control means 'losing it' totally.

There are many misconceptions about Alzheimer's: that you can't die from it, that only old people get it, that it simply makes you forget names and faces. I'm finding that having Alzheimer's for me has not really stopped me remembering names, places or faces. In fact people are sometimes amazed at my memory, but it is more for *past* events, not recent ones (and it takes effort and time). Rather, the disease affects so much more of my *daily* functioning, and yet I look so well because what's wrong with me is inside my head.

And even the way I function socially may not let you know there is anything drastically wrong with me, or that I may be only a few years away from needing full nursing care. I am adept at 'cover-up' strategies. I laugh and joke; I speak slowly so as to make sure I don't say silly words; I avoid questions; I try to cover up when my sentences aren't going the way I intended. I try so very hard for the short time I am with you that you would hardly know I was ill.

So much so do I succeed in this cover-up, that even my family doctor said: 'She's not that bad, at all. You'd hardly know she had Alzheimer's!' Indeed, every now and then the girls and I joke 'I'm so well, why don't I go back to work!' But of course we all know that is impossible, a pipedream.

After a social chat with you when I might have seemed so incredibly well and mentally focused, after you have gone I sink back exhausted, monosyllabic, wrung out and empty of all showmanship. It may take me at least a few hours lying down with my eyes closed to recover. My brain might be firing so much that later, at night, it simply will not switch off and let me sleep.

A migraine is also very likely – my brain's way of saying 'Enough!' Often I wish I only had Alzheimer's, without the migraines that seem to result from the effort I make to appear 'normal'. But I want to make the most of the time left to me, so the pain and illness is a side effect I'll just have to get used to.

And, of course, all of this assumes I am taking my tablets, the tacrine which I've been taking since October 1995. When I don't take them, and it is all too easy for me to forget them, then the world goes too fast for me to keep up. I can't even pretend to be 'normal'. I'm off-line, unable to speak or to think, lost in a foggy confusion. Ianthe describes how I look as: 'You just look absent, not there somehow.'

Chapter 8

From 'super-memory' to losing the plot

'Micheline, could you get the milk please?' I said, slowly and carefully, making sure the words came out right.

'Mum, I just got it! – I walked right past you just now.' She was annoyed with me, I could tell.

'Why can't I have a normal mother?' she was thinking. 'No-one else at school has to put up with this. They all tease me because my mum is demented, and they say I am going demented too! It's not fair!'

It's a far cry from the person I used to be. I always remembered everything, despite being super-fast: fast at reading, quick to ask questions, and always impatient to go on to the next topic. I came in the top two or three at school and at university. My intelligence level was high – indeed I did intelligence tests for fun, scoring anything between 150 and 200.

But I was also super-intolerant – other people were always so slow. Conversations even with brilliant scientists could be exasperating – how could they take so long to get the point! I had always to explain things that seemed so obvious to me. It was all too easy to do something myself rather than to wait until someone else could understand what they had to do.

I was always mystified as to how anyone could forget things – my own memory was like a giant, ever-changing and inter-connecting patchwork, or a huge hard drive, with many gigabytes of memory – a readily accessible parallel processor. Everything was immediately available for recall. I used to think that this was normal and everyone else who couldn't remember, or make connections between various memories and current events, must just not be trying very hard.

I could, for example, carry around in my head all the girls' needs, activities, all the household things, all the letters at home and at work I had received or needed to write, everyone's phone numbers (for work and home). I had no difficulty remembering my Medicare number (10 digits), my Visa card number (16 digits), tax file number, driver's licence number, health fund number and so on. I could fill out all forms without needing to refer to the original cards.

At work I remembered all the detail of scientific research I was shown on a visit, even years later if shown something else, when my brain would often make a lateral leap so that I could connect up the two areas of research and suggest that there might be advantage in cooperation. I would remember all the details of all the tasks my office of some thirty people was involved with, and also the directions I wanted to see us take. Often I would, in a meeting with staff, say 'But this and that happened'. Even if they did not remember it, they would always take my word for it, for my memory was known to be accurate.

Now, of course, I'm no longer such a 'super-memory', although my memory is still a lot better than might be expected. So much so that 'normal' people don't really notice anything wrong with my memory. But I do. It is shot to pieces, it is no longer as three-dimensional, and there are no longer those interconnections.

But how would I be now if I had started with a 'normal' memory before getting this disease?

Without a shopping list it is pointless me venturing to the shop.

Without my diary, I don't remember what day it is, what anyone is doing, where they are and so on. I don't seem to have space in my brain any more for that sense of 'Thursday-ness' (or whatever day it might happen to be), or 'April-ness', or '1998-ness'.

I'm finding this limits my ability to chat. I struggle to find the words in response to questions like 'how has your day been?' I usually have to think frantically to remember what day is it? – is it morning or afternoon? – what have I done today?!

Even more difficult is: 'Where are the girls today and how are they all?' I cannot remember when asked a question unexpectedly, and get even more stressed by the guilt that I can't remember where my girls are! Thank goodness I don't have any little children – they could get up to all sorts of mischief, and I wouldn't remember where I'd left the toddler!

So if you ask me a simple question, I am slow in responding while I search through my more limited and uni-dimensional data banks. It's as if, on a computer, I can't have more than one window open at once, or more than one application running. I have to 'open up' the window or application each time you ask about these things, so it takes more time.

I can be quite distracted, starting something, stopping, starting something else, unless I make a special effort to do only one thing at a time. If I lose this control, then I go on what my daughters call my 'frenzies' – just trying to do far too much all at once and not knowing when to stop. I infuriate my daughters because I often struggle on like this, without asking for help.

Wondering why I never ask for help, at first I thought 'Am I an incorrigible martyr?'

When I am busy with my frenzied task, I never think about anyone helping me, nor do I realise it is too much for me – until I finish and find I am too exhausted to do any more than sink into bed. It's because I simply don't remember that help is there to be had. Unless someone is right there beside me, I don't remember they are there, and could help. It sounds terrible to say this, but if my daughters are not at home, it is a big struggle to remember where they are, and their very existence doesn't really come to mind – unless I pass their bedroom, or see something belonging to them.

So I don't remember my neighbour is there, and we could go for a walk together; I don't remember that I could go for a walk myself; I don't think to ask for help in so many ways, because I forget that I am surrounded by friends only too glad to help if asked.

And therein lies the problem: how am I going to remember to ask!

I tax my family's patience so many times, because how I behave in just so many situations triggers in them quite normal emotional responses to someone else's 'bad behaviour'. Even I wonder at times why I can't be a little more 'normal'. But my behaviour comes from a disease process in my brain – I can't help it, however much I try.

Not only was I 'super-memory', but I always thought of myself as an 'in parallel' person – someone who can do several things at once. Indeed, I got irritated with anyone who did things methodically, one at a time. Now I'm slowly learning how to do things 'in series' – one after the other, slowly and carefully – and realising what an intolerant and difficult person I must have been for anyone not super-fast.

I realised I needed to change, to take into account my more limited brain power, when in late 1995, I was doing my chores in my usual way. I had put dinner on to cook, was putting a few loads of washing through the machine, and doing some ironing in between. Any busy working mother will relate to this being simply the 'survival mode' of getting everything done in the tiny snatches of time available between sleep and work. Even though I was by then a full-time mum, old habits die hard!

I was taking out the washing, when I smelled burning, and suddenly remembered dinner was cooking. I quickly put down the washing to rescue the dinner, but *en route* walked past the ironing board and realised I was in the middle of ironing too. Clearly I couldn't continue to do things in parallel if I completely forgot all the other tasks when I was doing just one of them. Either the house would burn down, the clothes would get ruined or dinner would have to be scraped into the bin.

It took a month or so to become comfortable with doing one thing at a time, but now it is the only way I can handle life, as I can simply always only remember the task I am currently doing. It's as if there is a much more limited filing space in my brain to hold different things in mind at the same time.

If I lose concentration momentarily during a task, I can get very confused and forget what I am supposed to be doing – even if it is the only thing I am attempting at the one time. This came home to me in late 1995, when I made a phone call to a roof tiler to arrange for him to fix my roof. During the time the phone was ringing I forgot who I was calling, and when someone answered 'Hello?', I had no idea who I was meant to be ringing, and of course got no clues from 'Hello?' So I had to mumble an apology and hang up – and that was only in the first few months after diagnosis!

Now, such events are commonplace in all sorts of tasks – and I become very tired quite quickly, from the effort of concentrating all my limited brain power on the task at hand.

Even if I try my hardest, events and phrases just disappear from my consciousness…my sieve brain leaks too much! There are simply huge gaps, where I don't register an event – the memory is not laid down anywhere in my brain. So it is not that I have forgotten and you can remind me. It is as if it never happened. Even if you tell me what happened, it means nothing to me. I'll just smile politely and try to pretend I remember all about it.

I picked up my eldest daughter one rainy evening, from her flat only two minutes away by car. This was a Tuesday evening – the next day, as usual, she would not be working and we would take this opportunity to have some time together. Well, as we drove away from her house I asked if she would need a lift to work the next day. She reminded me that she never worked on Wednesdays.

Then she proceeded, briefly, to describe the various chores she would do tomorrow, on her day off from work, and what we would do with our time together. Seconds later, as we drew into my garage, I asked if she needed a lift to work tomorrow. Luckily we can laugh about it.

When I watch TV, I often lose track of the plot because there are gaps everywhere in the storyline taken in by my brain. Presumably I am not retaining parts of the movie or whatever long enough in my short-term memory to get it transferred into my long-term memory and hence into an overall understanding of what is happening. Some parts I miss because there is too much happening at once on the screen or in the room around me, or if the people on TV are speaking too fast or not very clearly, or there is simply too much background noise or music happening at the same time as speech. I find now that I'm best watching things like wildlife programs, gardening and home- care shows. And adverts are definitely overload – we always mute these, and I look away from the TV if possible, for even the sights alone are much too confusing.

In prayer, I get muddled and vague, wandering off. I can hear you now, 'That always happens to me' – but it is now much more than when I was 'normal'; it happens all the time, even if I am not tired. So I find using the Prayer Book daily services is one way of really helping me focus my time with God.

Chapter 9

A confusion of sight and sound

I had got all dressed up to go out with my Bible study group to a restaurant one evening in late 1995. There were about twelve of us, around a big table, in a busy and large restaurant, with a pianist playing lovely background music. I should have really enjoyed the evening – great friends, good food, fun conversation, lovely music. But I didn't. I felt I was fading, the sounds were getting distant, faces were difficult to focus on, and I found it harder and harder to concentrate on what people were saying.

The party broke up and I walked across the car park, in the chill of the clear night air, to my car, trying to chat with a couple of my friends walking the same way to their car. I sank into the seat, and made it home, opened the garage door, drove in, got out, walked no further than my dining room and sank into the nearest chair. I just couldn't go any further, my head was ringing with noise, echoing around inside, my eyes felt tired and dry, my muscles felt non-existent.

Ianthe was sitting at the dining table, studying. She cried out 'Mum! What's wrong?' I hardly had the energy to reply, mumbling something like 'I'm just so terribly tired, can you help me upstairs to bed?' From that day on I refused invitations to noisy restaurants, and big groups of people, sticking to smaller places, quieter nights, and just a few friends.

Busy shopping centres are much less accessible to me, as I find them simply exhausting, with loud 'muzak', tills ringing, people talking, children crying. Even a quiet shopping trip can be very stressful if I go with someone, and am expected to hold a conversation as well as cope with the shopping decisions, and the sights and sounds around me.

It is like someone saying 'You will like my new compact discs. Here, I'll put three or four of them on at once so you can enjoy them.' It is just so hard, and takes so much effort to focus on the one source of sound that I am supposed to be listening to or responding to.

But church is OK, even if it is really noisy with loud music, because there is usually only one thing happening at a time. I can follow and take part easily, worshipping God. Bible study I can cope with too, as long as it remains focused on the study. The minute it breaks out into several different conversations, I can no longer deal with what is happening.

It's hard for me sometimes to understand what people are saying to me because I miss the first word or so, and cannot make sense of the rest of the sentence. This is particularly difficult on the phone, where there are no visual clues or a context to help me try to work out what the topic is.

For a year or so after diagnosis, I let my answering machine pick up the call, so that I knew who it was, and had time to work out what they were saying, before picking up the phone. But when people left messages on the answering machine, my daughters had to listen to them, for not only had I no idea who it was (too fast, doesn't sound like anyone I recognise etc.), but also I had no chance of capturing what the telephone number was, let alone writing it down.

I nearly wiped one message because I thought it was a wrong number – but when I asked Micheline to check it before we erased it, she said, 'Mum! That's my Dad wishing us a happy new year!'

I'm reluctant to answer the phone now, unless it is for exceptional circumstances, for it is difficult to work out who is speaking and what they are saying – particularly if there is background noise at their end, such as music or talking. Then I have just as much trouble getting words together in my head to make a sensible response fast enough. Words alone are the key to communicating by telephone, and now I need to rely on more time, more visual clues, more pantomime, to help my communication.

My church gave me a fax machine in April 1997 – it put me in touch with the world again! I can 'talk' to you at my speed, respond when I'm able to, and have time to understand what you 'say' to me. And I find that we write down much more than we would say, so I get much more amusing letters, full of anecdotes, and very meaningful words of love and encouragement.

I find it very difficult to tell where a sound is coming from, too. I am often startled by someone coming unexpectedly through a door, or look the wrong way to the miaow of a cat, and so on. I find it just as difficult to know what the sound actually is, and it takes me some time to process it. Instead of hearing a sound, and knowing what it is and where it is coming from as an automatic process, now I can almost chart the steps my brain is taking. A sound? Yes, a sound. Where from? Not sure. What is it? I can't tell.

One evening, I was very anxious about something I heard at my back door and peered into the gloom of the crisp winter dusk. But I couldn't sort out the shadow in the garden from reflections in the glass door. I had a few moments of panic before finally Ianthe said, 'It's only me, Mum!' There she was, shivering, I could see her clearly now, standing out there in the cold waiting to be let in!

I tend to overreact – in my daughters' eyes – getting too anxious or startled at sudden sounds. But to me the sounds are very unfamiliar, strange, and stressful until I recognise what they are.

One evening I was with my daughters and a couple of their friends, watching videos. Suddenly I realised water was hammering in the pipes. This usually meant that the corporate body watering system was on. But somehow I got it into my mind that it meant my own watering system had broken down and water was probably gushing over my garden. Once I have an idea in my head, I have mental 'blinkers' on and cannot properly perceive and assess my environment as sights and sounds get very muddled up. I rushed outside in my socks, and got wet feet, and then raced back inside saying, in a panicky voice, 'The watering system is flooding all over the garden!'

Ianthe came out to look, and gently led me in. 'Mum, it's raining!'

I find that my peripheral vision shrinks if I am in a busy place. It's as if my brain self-limits the number of sights it can cope with. So I can't see what is happening around me, and get lost or confused easily. It's as if I have blinkers on.

A friend came over to help me take cuttings and plant them. A restful activity, you might think. But no, my brain was simply not dealing very well with the array of cuttings we had taken, the pots on the table, the bucket of soil, the hormone to dip shoots into, the pile of discarded leaves, the secateurs, and so on. We were doing all of this at normal speed (I think), and probably what I would once have thought of as extremely slow. But my brain was cutting out things in the field of view, which by now was limited to just the table in front of me. So it was harder for me to locate items, as well as carry out the actions I was meant to be doing.

When I am bombarded with sight or sound, I get what the girls call my vague look – and they can all do a very amusing imitation of it! This is basically when my brain has reached the overload stage and has simply cut out, and there is no energy or resource left in me to cope with what's going on around me. Often, if I don't find somewhere quiet very quickly, a migraine may follow.

The noisy environment seems to reverberate inside my head, and it just gets too confusing for my brain to be able to sift out any sense from what I hear. The world suddenly becomes remote, distant and disconnected from me. I feel worn out, wrung out, and desperate to lie down with my eyes closed. Or, as I put it to my girls, 'I'll just go somewhere quiet and stare blankly into space for a while.' We actually say 'Bare stankly', as we're keen on spoonerisms at our place! I'm sure it's a good brain exercise for me to try to understand them and to make them up – and amazingly I'm still quite good at it!

The reason for the blank stare of many Alzheimer's patients may well be that they have been exposed to too much stimulus, so there would be little point, and indeed it may be quite counterproductive, to try to 'jolly them out of it' by more stimulus, whether visual or sound.

Chapter 10

A jumble of words

We were sitting around the dinner table and I was talking about the time I had broken my arm as a little girl, and Ianthe asked, 'How old were you then?' I said, 'I was half past four', then paused, realising something was not quite right, just before we all broke out into gales of laughter.

Finding words in my head, even when I'm initiating conversation and not trying to respond to questions, is very difficult – and often something stupid like that comes out. Sometimes I simply give up on what I am trying to say, because the words just can't come to mind fast enough for me to be able to speak at an acceptable rate, and I'm worried I'll say something silly.

Often I draw little pictures in the air when words fail me or use quite innovative analogies, such as: 'that bottle lying on its flat in the fridge' to describe a bottle on its side. Or I call the mail box 'that box you put letters in with stamps on them'. All of this is usually accompanied by a visual pantomime of gestures to give further clarity (or entertainment value) to what I want to communicate. And that makes it almost impossible on the phone, because you just can't see this pantomime!

If you are suggesting something to me, I cannot respond quickly with clear reasoning as to why I might not be able to do it, and even if I manage this, you'll have ready a list of clear reasons why I should. This results in me often going along with what someone else wants to do, because it is just too hard to explain why I might prefer something else. So I am 'pressured', even by well-meaning family and friends, into situations that are stressful for me.

I can understand how Alzheimer's patients might become quite violent when hurried or harried along by well-meaning carers, because they have pent-up frustration inside at simply being unable to get the words out – 'I don't want to do this!' and to tell you why not.

Before this disease, I would be frustrated because I couldn't speak as fast as my brain could process ideas, thoughts, solutions. Often it was almost as if my brain would say: 'Come on mouth – keep up with me!' Now the opposite is true, and my mouth waits impatiently, 'er-ing' and 'um-ing', until finally some words come through from the brain.

The jumble of words inside my 'treacle brain' feels as if shelves of neatly ordered words in my head, all filed appropriately according to subject and so on, have been swept to the floor and are lying there in muddled heaps for me to sort through and try to find the one that belongs to what I am trying to say.

Just imagine waking up one day, and trying to speak and finding somehow words have disappeared mid-sentence – vanished without a trace. You know you are trying to say a sentence and have a 'gut-feel' as to its meaning as a whole, but important component parts are missing. Slowly your mouth waits, your fogged brain struggles, and sometimes the right word (or something reasonably close to it) shapes itself and you carefully, slowly say it, checking it's right.

If you don't concentrate, you know something stupid will come out.

- One evening Rhiannon wanted me to open the car boot so she could put in her horse gear. While she asked me this, I was first of all thinking – why does she want the boot open? – and then gazed blankly at the passenger seat next to me. So I said, 'What will you do if I open the car seat?'

- Another evening I was in the kitchen preparing roast dinner, when I noticed a saucepan was boiling over. I needed Rachel to take it off the heat quickly, but quickly is not something my brain recognises as a mode of operation nowadays – let alone coming up with the right words. So I yelled, 'It's going like bananas!'

- On her birthday, Micheline was rushing around the house doing a treasure hunt Ianthe had prepared, and a clue was hidden up in the smoke detector. I said, 'Get the tissue!' (to stand on, instead of the stool).

And now, imagine this is happening to you nearly *every* time you speak – and you know it's probably going to get worse. Often you wonder whether it's worth trying to speak, because it always comes out wrong and everyone laughs at you.

That's what it's like to have Alzheimer's.

And it's the same with writing. You are writing a short note slowly and carefully, but you look over what you have just written and there are quite a few letters missing, and those that are there are shaped peculiarly. You look over the words and see bits missing – an 's' here, a 't' there – and you see strange joins between letters that make the letters a bit illegible.

What's happening to the link between my brain and hand? Why can I bash away at the computer, but struggle to write a few words in a wobbly and childlike hand? Is it because you need to remember how to form the letters, as well as remember what you want to write, how to spell the word, and in what order the words have to be written to make sense?

Maybe this is why writing on the computer is much easier, even though I learned that only relatively recently compared to writing by hand. (With Alzheimer's, apparently what you learned last goes first.) Each letter only requires one key stroke, and not any memory of how to form it, and of course there is that wonderful spellcheck, and ability to correct, insert and whatever later on. But even then, there are those awful moments when I struggle to remember whether it is 'right' or 'write', 'there' or 'their' – very scary for someone who was always so critical of others' spelling and grammar.

The doctors can't say why this is happening or what else to expect, because for each patient, their brain is wired up differently, and the disease is progressing through that wiring in a slightly different way for each person. So you never know what to expect next.

Then there is reading out loud. I can still read silently very quickly – not quite so super abnormally fast as I used to, but still a lot faster than many other 'normal' people. So the world of books is still very accessible to me, a wealth of enjoyment to dip into and savour. But I can't get my mouth to work at normal speeds, when reading out aloud.

So in church, I find it difficult to join in with the rest of the congregation when we read out parts of the responses in the service. I am way too slow. They're 'amening' when I'm a few words or so behind! I suppose there is just too much brain processing needed to see the words, understand them individually, make sense of them in context, then send all that back to speaking centres, so that I can formulate the right sounds, with the right inflection.

I tire very easily, simply because of the effort required to get through what others would think of as quiet and relaxing days, but for me are periods of bombardment with a range of stimuli, and huge amounts of effort just to say a simple sentence. When I am tired, I feel, and sound, like a clockwork toy whose mechanism has run down; or, as Micheline said once, 'You are sounding like a robot, Mum. Let's stop talking now.' I speak very slowly, and sentences become stuck midway as I grasp for words, as if my flow of ideas is now paddling through thick treacle.

But I wonder how bad I would be by now if I hadn't started with such a high level of verbal skills to start with? Would I be almost mute?

Back in 1984, when I did the Princeton University Graduate Management Admission Test, I scored on the 99 percentile for my verbal skills, simply meaning that I was in the top 1 per cent of the world.

Growing up bilingual (English/Dutch) also challenged my verbal skills. And we delighted in Scrabble, travelling between the two countries clutching Scrabble letters for the two languages, tossing up to see in what language we would play. Then the competition would intensify, to see who got the highest score, and we would try to better our record for overall game score. My family are still 'Scrabbling' – even my grandma at nearly 103! I tried in 1996, playing a game in English with my mother, but I am no longer in their league.

So I am drawing on every remaining ounce of that earlier capability now, as I struggle to communicate at an acceptable pace with the rest of my now quite small world.

Chapter 11

Life's essentials

The most essential of all my essentials is my tacrine – this drug keeps me going at the rate at which everyone else functions, so I can keep up with you, follow what you say, and try to respond. Basically, it bathes my brain in lots of chemical messenger, so that what's left up there works as best it can. When I don't take it, I experience a foggy confusion, a deep restlessness and a feeling of exhaustion – often my head aches around the eyes and temples, and all I want to do is sleep. I can't understand what is happening around me because you are all going too fast. I cut out, and just look emptily at my surroundings, not really following what is going on.

My 'beeping pill box' is another of life's essentials, reminding me to take my tacrine. It once belonged to Karen's father. He had Parkinson's and Alzheimer's diseases, and died in late 1995. Each morning my routine is to put the tablets in the various compartments and to set the timer. But if my routine is disturbed, such as on holidays or when the girls are home from school, this can easily be forgotten. I've been known to leap up suddenly in the evening and cry out 'Oops! My tablets! I've not taken any all day!'

The pill box can be programmed to beep when it is time to take tablets, and beeps loud and clear for long enough to be found if, as sometimes happens, I have mislaid it. The girls get embarrassed if it beeps in public, because if there are other noises in my environment I cannot distinguish the beeping. So there are often cries of 'Mum! Your pill box. It's beeping!'

When I focus attention to listen for the beep, of course I can hear it. There is nothing wrong with my hearing, only my ability to filter noises from my environment. But then, often, I assiduously open the pill box to find that I have forgotten to put my day's tablets in there, even though I have obviously set it to beep when tablet time comes round!

My diary is an important essential, with my routine tasks carefully listed and 'measured out in easy instalments' throughout the week. I refer to it frequently, so as to remind myself which day it is, and what I have undertaken (to myself) to do for the day. If I don't parcel out activities such as cleaning, gardening and washing during the week, I go into 'frenzy' mode and try to do everything at once, working myself to the point of exhaustion – and of course to withdrawal, where I sit with my blank stare, unable to initiate activity or to participate in what seems to be frenetic activity all around me. And then this is usually followed by a migraine, my brain's way of telling me to stop being so stupid!

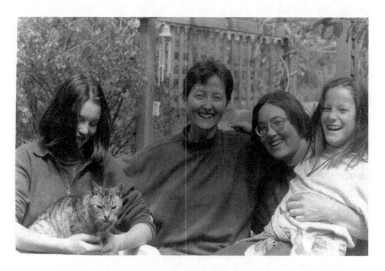

*First Christmas after diagnosis in 1995; Christine
and her girls happy in their garden*

Really, the diary was the most important present I could have had for Christmas 1995, with a day to a page and plenty of space to list jobs and note times to collect and deliver the girls to various activities, in the course of running 'Mum's taxi service'. Another was given to me for Christmas 1996. Both had beautiful covers made from my daughters' paintings, and were carefully covered in clear plastic so that they survived life in the kitchen – on the breadbin, where I keep lists, keys and the like. I wonder what would happen if someone moved the breadbin!

Routine is vital. I have developed not only routine tasks for the week, but also fixed places to put things (such as the immovable breadbin!). I'm sure even those who are blessed with a full complement of brain cells could benefit from more certain storage places. Even before my illness I often misplaced items. The difference now is that unless an item is in the place where I always put it, I will *always* forget where it is, and there is *no* chance of me remembering where I have put it. Every so often I go on searches of the complete house, garage, car and garden when I have not put something in its usual place, because of being distracted by, say, someone telling me something, or a noise outside. These searches are exhausting, and very frustrating because even when I find the object, I have no recollection of how it got there.

'Brain gym' is an essential. It is important, according to my specialist, to keep my brain active. I used to say to my girls, when they didn't want to read a book, do homework or play maths games, that the brain is just like our muscles and needs regular exercise to keep it in top form. Now, in my reading about the brain, I have found out that brain cells can keep trying to make new connections to overcome damage, as long as you keep challenging them to do things. Brain gym, then, is keeping those cells on their toes, reaching out to each other every time a pathway between them is damaged.

With books, I need an absolutely quiet environment (not always easy with daughters in and out of the house), and then to keep re-reading parts until I have a firm hold of the plot, and to read in as large chunks as possible so that I haven't forgotten too much of the plot by the time I return to reading once more. I have also started to take notes of key characters, places and events, to review each time I take up the book again. At least a book goes at my pace, which could be slow or even slower depending on how tired I am.

I read lots of detective novels when I was on sick leave at first, relishing the time to do this – and I was always completely enthralled until the very last page, as usually I could not remember from one reading session to the next the names or significance of the various characters!

Now I am trying to read more 'worthwhile' books. If I've only got a limited amount of time left to be able to read, I want to make that time count. But when anyone asks me what book I am reading, or what is it about, of course I am usually lost for words – but I can tell them that I am enjoying it immensely!

For me, another essential to keep me from 'frenzy' mode, is 'purr therapy'. This term was coined by Karen's husband, Roger, to describe the therapeutic value of sitting with a purring cat on your lap. I have found that cats have become a very important part of my life now, as they keep me calm, and stop me racing around trying to do too much at once. They give me 'brain time out' as I sit quietly stroking them and just sitting, doing nothing.

When our 20-year-old cat died in late 1996 I was really devastated, and found that I had regressed considerably in the space of less than a week. I had many more episodes of being unable to muster my thoughts in order to speak even a sentence or two, and I was beset by migraines and exhaustion. And, of course, I was deprived of time to sit idly with a cat purring on my lap.

Our house felt so empty without our faithful friend, and we only managed to last four days before going to the animal refuge and choosing two cats of character: one is a tabby who is quite fat and has a rapid, breathless purr. He thinks he is a dog, wears a leather-studded collar, and follows us around, even sitting when told to do so. We have called him Chunkers, to suit his spreading girth and hearty appetite. The other is a timid long-haired female, with a soft relaxing purr. She is slender and graceful, despite a damaged leg, and we call her Willow. The following year Chunkers moved out to live with Ianthe – there was a personality conflict with Willow – and we added two lively but very 'purry' kittens to our menagerie. Now I have a choice of several forms of purr therapy!

I have asked that if I need to go to a nursing home, could it be one that allows cats, as I am sure I will continue to need purr therapy.

I discovered another one of life's new essentials for me when I travelled to Europe with Ianthe to visit my family in 1996 – earplugs! They mute the confusion of sounds and give me a new perspective:

> Waiting in a quiet area of the airport I am revelling in the newfound joy of earplugs. I sit as if isolated from all around me, with all sounds muted, muffled, distant – feeling like a deep-sea diver – watching aeroplanes and trucks on the tarmac, as restful and hushed as if they were tropical fish. No more struggling to keep up with a busy, multi-tracked, conflicting and confusing world. What a blessing Ianthe is. I can sit remote, detached, disengaged, whilst she steers us, organises us, and takes charge, shepherding me carefully through this airport chaos in my tropical aquarium bubble!

For Ianthe, she commented:

> So far so good, we've checked in for our international flight. Mum has sunk into the reverie of the earplug world, taking her mind with her. Her vague look is constant, but without that edge of fatigue.

So now earplugs are very helpful if I am to visit a busy shopping centre, or anywhere else with lots of background noise.

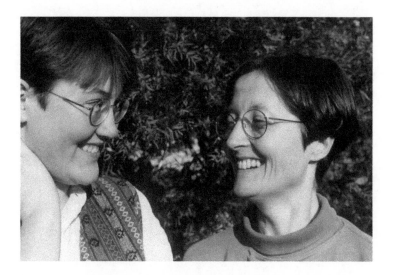

Ianthe and Christine in 1996 before going overseas

If you were to ask me what are the most important things to help me now, in this stage of the disease, I'd say tacrine and brain gym. They keep me functioning, and keep challenging my brain to function, hopefully delaying my deterioration – and keeping me clinging to that precipice by my fingernails!

An adventure into the unknown

Chapter 12

Trying to be prepared

Should I renew subscriptions to the newspaper, to my Bible study text – will I still be able to read for the rest of this year? Should I still try to do my finances and my tax return, or will I make mistakes without knowing it?

It is an interesting adventure, this Alzheimer's, because no-one can predict what functions I will lose or when. And because of my scientific training, I feel I have a unique opportunity to live my own experiment – and to record what is happening to me in the hope it may give some insight into this 'brain-rot', as I have called it in some of my darker moments.

The ability to calculate can be lost quite early on in the disease, and can then result in some financial difficulty if the Alzheimer's sufferer is also the 'finance manager' for the household and won't admit to any difficulty. At some stage, soon, presumably I will lose my understanding of what numbers are, what they mean, and what you do with them. Every now and then, this is already happening, as I write down a number for my bank balance, against expenses, and struggle to recall what to do, whether and how to subtract one from the other.

So I am already showing my daughters the way in which I keep track of finances, including the spreadsheet I use for budgeting. They are all now practising with their own finances – which in itself is a good thing. But I am trying to keep calculating something, however trivial, every few days or so, as part of my brain gym – for I do find that if I don't look at numbers for a while, it takes more and more effort to remember what they all mean.

As I mentioned, writing by hand has become very difficult. I had certainly heard of other Alzheimer's sufferers who had lost the ability to write, even to sign their name, quite early on in their illness. Although this disease follows a unique course in every individual, and it was always possible I would retain this ability for quite some time, I didn't want to wake up one day and find that I could no longer sign my name on cheques or Visa card slips.

So, only a few months after diagnosis, I arranged for Ianthe (who fortunately was over the age of eighteen, and able to take this on) to have general power of attorney. This was arranged so that although I could continue to act on my own behalf, she could also do so at any time now or in the future and, in 'legalese': 'This Power of Attorney is given with the intention that it will continue to be effective notwithstanding that after its execution I suffer loss of capacity through unsoundness of mind.' This certainly gave me peace of mind. It means she can already act on my behalf, whenever necessary.

Having a disease which slowly takes away your mind bit by bit makes you realise how important it is to hang onto those few freedoms you already have for as long as possible (such as driving, or operating your finances), because the world out there is only too willing to take those freedoms away from you. If I make a common mistake, it is seen as being of much more significance than if others make the same mistake – it is seen as yet more evidence of me 'losing it', and therefore of needing to be stopped from doing things, or to be overly protected when going about life's normal business. As yet, I still have enough capacity to protest loudly if others try to read into my actions more than they would into similar actions by a 'normal' person!

Chapter 13

My car's an alien spaceship! – and other oddities

In mid-1996 I started having difficulty when I first sat in the car to drive. I just couldn't remember what pedal was supposed to do what, and where I was meant to put my feet. Also backing out of the garage was often challenging, remembering which way to steer when going backwards.

But it always came back to me very quickly, so that my passengers were not aware of my problems. That was until later in 1996, when I had driven Rhiannon to the paddock to put her horse, Arthur, in his stable. I was helping her with various wholesome outdoor activities, such as cleaning out Arthur's stable, fetching more hay with the wheelbarrow, and getting his feed ready for the night.

It was dusk before we got back into the car, about forty-five minutes after our arrival at the stables. But in that forty-five minutes, my car had been transformed into an alien spaceship! I sat in the driver's seat completely confused. What was I meant to do with my hands, and where on earth was I meant to put my feet down there in the gloom of the car floor? It felt as if I had never sat in anything like this machine before.

'Um, er,' I said, 'could you shine the torch down there at my feet a moment?' I fumbled with my hands on the wheel, adjusted my seating position, while desperately trying to remember which pedal was what. 'Where do I put my feet? What's that little pedal there in the corner?'

Rhiannon, who at that time had not even got her learner's licence, had to take me patiently through where I was to put my feet and my hands, and which pedal did what. We drove off very slowly, over the paddock roads, with a few stutters now and then while I rapidly re-learned my driving procedures. But it all came back quickly – as if it had never been forgotten.

We laughed over the irony of it all – Rhiannon having to teach her mum to drive, when that was what I was supposed to do for her in a few months' time! But deep inside I was scared. Was this what it was going to be like? Was it all starting to happen now? What would I forget next? For a month or so, I was very uncertain, very cautious, and anxious in everything I did, just wondering whether that sudden feeling of being somewhere so totally alien would happen again.

I was very careful whilst driving, focusing on each and every action, not listening to the radio or having any conversations, and going at speeds well within my own limits, and well back from any cars ahead. I travelled on familiar routes, at quiet times, and never in the dark. Canberra, where I live, is very fortunate in having excellent roads and very little traffic, so it provided me with the ideal driving environment.

In April 1997, I stopped driving. It was getting too stressful and tiring, and I would often worry that I would not see things I should have done, because of difficulties with my peripheral vision. The busy roads would somehow trigger my brain into limiting its input, so I had a narrower field of view the busier the traffic got – definitely not good for anybody's safety! Road works worried me too, as I could not react fast enough to suddenly changed road instructions, and would become confused as to where I was and which way to go.

The girls go off to school now each day by bus, and I am finding it much easier to cope with a more slowly paced and quieter day, without the stress of working hard to remember how to drive, where and when to go, and how to react to traffic and changed road conditions.

There are other oddities, other unexpected things; no-one can warn me what will happen, or if something happens, explain why it does. So I often stumble over my own feet – but why? I need to keep focused on the task of climbing the stairs or walking over uneven ground, because if I try to do this as well as something else, like talk, I stumble over my own feet. I can't talk and walk up stairs at the same time, I 'can't walk and chew gum'!

My emotions seem a little awry. Sometimes I am a bit more teary than before, for no apparent reason. But more often I seem to have what feels like a sort of emotional blank, which to my daughters looks like a lack of sparkle, of charisma. I don't get as excited as I used to, and I just feel a little 'flat'. It takes too much energy to react with emotion: where once it seemed automatic, now it takes actual mental effort to consider a situation, and then how to react to it.

Every now and then I smell things – nice things, nasty things – which aren't really there, and are totally unrelated to what is around me. Most odd, and a bit disconcerting. Sometimes, too, this smell from nowhere also triggers a whole string of memories for me.

I have an annoying twitch in my eyelid which started in 1997 – I can hear you now: 'I have that all the time!' But do you really? I have this twitch non-stop, and it occurs so often that it is very intrusive. So much so, I thought I would count them one day. And between 9 p.m. one day and 9 p.m. the next I had twenty-eight eye twitches lasting from just ten or so minutes at a stretch, to nearly an hour long. The specialist couldn't explain it, saying it usually happened to young nervous people. I'm certainly not young, and I'm not nervous.

So why does it happen? And why does it sometimes not happen quite so frequently? Are my nerves simply getting a bit confused, what with all the tangles and so on in my brain?

Chapter 14

From 'super-mum' to dependent mum

One evening Rhiannon was really upset about an argument with Micheline, and how I had reacted. She wrote me a note about how unfair it all was, and how she felt everyone was against her and so on. I had obviously failed her – but I was so tired, so exhausted at trying to deal with mothering, when I was finding even just thinking and speaking to be so hard, so I wrote a note back:

> It's not fair to treat someone who is sick in the head as if she's normal, and if she wants things done, or wants to do something, or whatever, to stress her out so that she gets sicker. I can't help the way I behave – I'm sick in the head – and I can't carry on being this 'happy mother' act. I'm not happy. I'm stressed and I wish I could die more quickly so you didn't have to put up with me.

I had reached rock bottom – I could not do the thing I wanted to do most, and that was to restore my daughter's self-esteem, to reassure her of my love, to bring peace to the household. I really felt at that time that it would be better to die quickly than to suffer this prolonged illness, causing stress to my daughters.

At work, as a single mum, I found it busy, even frenetic, but somehow I managed to cope with a huge range of things in the office, as well as find time to be with my girls at home – to try to talk about their problems, their joys, their successes.

I never did the usual things of 'mothering' very well. I never owned more than one or two cookbooks, and the cupboards were often bare, as I had not had time to shop. Often we would have toast for dinner. The house was usually untidy and a bit grubby, because I had not had time to clean, and there were never enough clean clothes because I could really only get to washing, cleaning and shopping at weekends. I used to call ours a 'feral' household, because the girls would make gruesome food concoctions for themselves when they got home from school, and our house was often without all the home comforts many other people take for granted.

But what little time I did have, I tried to spend talking or listening to my girls – to me that was more important than all these other things. Ianthe has often said she always knew she was my real priority, even though I was away travelling, or away at work, or working at the computer at home.

Now I find, once again, I can do so little mothering, but now it's because I become exhausted very quickly, and can only operate relatively slowly if it involves talking and listening. It has become so hard to try to carry on caring for a 16- and an 11-year-old – to deal with their arguments, their needs, their cleaning, cooking, shopping, washing.

My greatest difficulty was simply that the house was too busy for me. There was too much going on, too much talking, too much activity, for me to keep up with. In particular, I had no resources left to deal with arguments, and tantrums or fights.

I look well, so why can't I be a 'normal' mother? I try my best, but it takes so much effort just to keep on top of daily routines, that the normal demands of my daughters rock me to the core and cause me lots of stress. I can't function well with 'surprises', spontaneity – sudden requests to take some daughter here or there, or to sign this form or that, or to look at this work or that, cause me great difficulty.

Most Alzheimer's sufferers, even the early-onset ones, don't have to deal with – and they usually have a partner to support them all this and their illness too. Usually their children have left home and they only have their own needs to deal with – and they usually have a partner to support them. I do wish I had got this disease when I was just a bit older, as Micheline is only twelve, and it is possible that I could need full nursing care before she finishes school.

But I want to make the most of my time with my girls, and not to waste time and emotional resources regretting what I might miss, like seeing their eventual career paths, cuddling any grandchildren and so on. To regret this would be to take away enjoyment from what I do have – and that is the time to be with them now. I want to make sure that all the brain power I have left goes into being with my daughters: listening to them, talking with them, and just letting them know I love them unconditionally. No matter what they have done, or no matter what their behaviour, I love them and want to be with them.

I want to be able to answer the really important questions, like 'Mum, will there be a McDonald's in heaven?', which Micheline has asked. And not just questions like where are my socks (how would I know!).

I also want to be able to treasure, to savour, little gifts they give me that mean just so much. Like the words on gift cards: 'Thanks for being a cool mum' and 'Thank you for always being there for me'.

So Rhiannon moved in mid-1997 to live nearby with Ianthe and Rachel. This takes a lot of the pressure off me, particularly reducing the busyness of the house. I can then give Micheline what mothering I can, while I can. I will still see Ianthe and Rhiannon most days, to share special times, to talk and to listen. I can see them at times when I am not tired, so I can muster the energy to be as much a 'proper mum' as possible.

They will all be able to take care of me – check the inevitable tablet box, check I have eaten, that I have food in the house, don't get 'frenzied' and so on. All of this will let me and my girls enjoy each day as it comes, and leave me free to use the brain I have left on the really important things in life – my daughters, loving them, knowing them, and being with them.

Chapter 15

A scary road ahead?

I'm beginning, I think, to get a sneak preview of some of the scary things that might lie ahead.

I was gardening on a beautiful sunny afternoon, a Saturday in late 1996. Crouching down, sweating and labouring in the hot sunshine, I had accumulated a small pile of weeds. I was thirsty, tired and aching everywhere, but I was determined to get this weeding done! All of a sudden I was somewhere else, with people chattering around me, and it was almost as if I was at a lively party. I shook my head, tried to see clearly the yellow weeding tool in my hand, and turned to a new patch of garden. But it happened again. And again, and again.

At last I went in, unsteadily, and Micheline came up to me and said, 'What's wrong, Mum?'

'I feel a bit peculiar, I'll just go and lie down, could you get me a glass of water?' I lay on the bed, but each time I relaxed, those chattering sights and sounds came again.

I went to the doctor on the Monday. She thought it was a reaction to some new tablets she had given me, so I stopped taking them, and the problem stopped.

But in March 1997 it all started happening again. And I was taking no new tablets. I was having quite a lot of migraines, and taking my usual migraine medication, but nothing new. I would just be drifting off to sleep, when I would be dragged awake, my body pushed down on the bed, or my jaw locked. I would see people sitting there with me, people talking, moving about me. But the really awful thing was that I was not asleep. I could not wake up and leave the nightmare behind. It was right there with me.

I would drift off finally to sleep, exhausted, but wake up at 12, at 1, at 1:40, at 2:30, at 4:15, at 7. Each time I awoke, I was in the middle of a vivid experience, pulling me this way and that. I felt bodily movement, falling, pulling, dipping, turning. I was hoarse from trying to speak, aching from trying to move. If only these were nightmares, I could wake up, but I was awake when they were happening.

When I told the specialist in April, he said I was probably now very sensitive to drugs, even my usual migraine tablets, given that there is less brain for them to work on.

He also made some comment about menopause. But my periods are still as regular as clockwork, and just the same as ever – indeed, this is quite a worry for me: what if I am still having periods if I need full nursing care and can no longer look after myself? Now my family doctor has reassured me, saying that when the time comes, she can give me a series of injections to induce menopause.

As I had experienced so many migraines over the past few months before seeing the specialist, up to two per week, he changed the migraine preventative medication. But the following week then became one of the worst I have ever experienced! Perhaps the new tablets may have triggered this whole series of exhausting hallucinatory nights. I dreaded the night, and dragged myself wearily through the days. I was absolutely exhausted by the time Saturday evening came round.

Ianthe asked me anxiously, 'You won't want to go to church tomorrow?'

I said, 'I'm too sick *not* to go to church! I need prayer.' Even though during those long nights I always felt that God was right there beside me in the midst of this suffering, I just wanted extra support for the terrible things happening to me as my brain seemed to be misfiring and tricking me.

That very Sunday, as I sat wearily on the pew, Brian, a member of our congregation, stood up and said that he felt we needed to pray for the gift of healing in our church. So I took him at his word, and after the service asked him, his sister, Pauline, and another friend, Helen, to pray for me after church, briefly explaining the problem. The prayer was great – none of that 'casting out demons' stuff – I certainly didn't feel my problem was anything spiritual, and would have felt most offended had it been suggested! I knew that it was just the physical damage to my brain reacting in a very odd way to the presence of yet another drug in my system.

That night was the first for a week where nothing 'odd' happened, and I actually got a few hours' sleep. It seems to have settled down now, and gradually I am building up my sleep resources, with only the occasional odd episode. But I do feel a little anxious, about just how little it might take to trip me over the edge again into a lot more of those hallucinations.

Who knows what will happen as my brain continues to deteriorate? But I am so glad I have faith to cling to. How would I cope without it?

Where to now?

Chapter 16

Our fifteen minutes of fame

An excuse I used back in 1996 for not getting on with writing this book was our appearance in other media, namely newspaper and TV – but that in itself acted as a prompt to me to get on with it, as my writing a book was mentioned in both.

It was Andy Warhol who said everyone has fifteen minutes of fame in their lives. For us it was in June–July of 1996. It all started with a joke item by Simon Grose in *The Canberra Times* about Ronald Reagan, headed 'Who's Al Zeimer?' I was appalled. As I had known Simon during my career in CSIRO and in the public service, I wrote a letter explaining that having Alzheimer's disease was no joke, that younger people can get it, and that it is about as tasteful as a joke about cancer to poke fun at the fading faculties of those with Alzheimer's. I suggested that he might want to do a feature on the disease, to raise awareness.

A few weeks later I got a call from Simon to express his deep regrets, and to let me know that the newspaper was interested in doing an article, and that a colleague of his, Verona Burgess, would be in touch. I thought no more of it until Verona rang me to make a time to come and see me. We eventually met after a series of migraines had delayed our meeting for a couple of weeks. She was sensitive and caring, and had already researched the topic well. I felt very comfortable sharing my story with her.

Only days later, expecting a feature on the disease with perhaps a few highlights from our discussion as an illustration, I was stunned to see a full-page feature on me, accompanied by a huge photo. However uncomfortable that made me feel – it really ruined my Saturday morning breakfast in bed! – I felt it was important to 'go public' and not be ashamed of my steadily growing disability, and to let others know just how much my faith sustains me in all of this. I still get occasional letters and cards from people who have seen the article, and have also been told by several friends that it resulted in quite a lot of discussion in various workplaces, as people come to grips with the need to understand that Alzheimer's is a physical disease, not a mental illness.

And here, I thought, the matter would end, and I could try to get back to normal. But a few days later, I had just got the girls off to school and was about to sip my freshly made cup of tea when the phone rang. It was a researcher from *A Current Affair*, Channel 9, asking if they could feature my family on their program. I said I'd need a day or so to think it over. I then rang a few friends to pray about it, and prayed with the girls too. We all felt it was the right thing to do, so I rang back and agreed to go ahead. I knew our church would be praying for us, and for the show, and felt confident we could leave it in God's hands.

The four-man crew (interviewer, producer, camera man and sound man) were friendly, compassionate and caring, while also being very professional and talented in their work. They spent two days with us, interviewing me and the girls, covering aspects of my daily routine, as well as shots of me writing at the computer – and, as is usual, making terrible typing errors – thank God for spellcheck!

They also flew Ianthe and me up to Sydney for some psychometric tests. I agreed to do this, as it is clear people (for example, my superannuation company) have a concept of these tests as being more like intelligence tests, or more complex material such as offered in management courses and the like. In reality these tests are more akin to preschool work, and demonstrate quite vividly how basic abilities become increasingly impaired in the progress of Alzheimer's.

The show went to air in July 1996, and was very good in covering the main aspects of Alzheimer's and its impact on our family. But many of our friends immediately spotted the essential ingredient that had been left out – all mention of our faith, and the place of God and our church 'family' in our lives, had been omitted.

The week following the program I gave the following talk at church:

> Thank you for all your prayers about the *A Current Affair* program.
>
> Well, I was confused and disappointed the evening of the program because all mention of our faith and of you wonderful people was cut out. I prayed the night after the program, saying 'I gave it to you, committed the production team and the editing to you, so why did you let it all get cut out? Did I get it wrong? I didn't get sick doing the program, so that part of our bargain worked out – but maybe I need not have gone through all of that? Was it really for you that we did it?'
>
> The next morning I was still quite down, when the phone rang. It was the interviewer, Mike Munro, ringing to ask if I liked the show. I said it was great, 'but the most important part, the central reason for our family being able to be happy – our faith and the people at our church – was omitted. Anyone who knows us will be puzzled.' He apologised profusely, and then said that their switchboard had been jammed with positive calls for two hours after the show went to air. Even Alzheimer's sufferers and their families had rung to say it had encouraged them and given them hope.
>
> He said that because of all this interest, the TV station management had asked him to do a one-hour special over the next year or so, and if we agreed, he would give me his personal guarantee that our

faith and our church would be very much part of the follow-up, and that they might even film us at church. Well, I certainly 'ate humble pie' in prayer afterwards. God did have it in hand after all, and the show, without any mention of faith, was drawing in people who wanted to hear more – maybe the TV special would be able to reach so many more people. Please keep praying, for God is in charge and we must not doubt him, but just wait to see how his will will be done!

After the first program, I got many letters and cards. Some of them touched us deeply, being wonderfully compassionate and open-hearted, generous in offers of help whenever needed. And we got more after the second program, filmed in February and screened in April 1997.

Three, in particular, I treasured: Rhiannon's day-care mother, who had looked after her from birth to preschool, wrote to me, telling me of her ongoing battle with multiple sclerosis; a lovely Anglican lady who was also being tested for Alzheimer's got in touch; and a distraught lady going through the trauma of diagnosis and coping with the disbelief of friends and family also wrote a long letter to me. We are all still in touch.

And one evening, Ianthe went to a cricket function and met her former coach and his wife. This lady was clearly having memory problems, so much so that they showed up in conversation over dinner. But she was now on tablets that would cure this in a matter of time. And this cure was as the result of watching the program!

They had seen the first program, realised that maybe something was really wrong, not just old age, and finally decided to see a doctor. The doctor had also seen the program, so took this very seriously and did all the tests possible to see if the memory problems were indeed the result of Alzheimer's, or of something curable. This one cure alone was, for us, worth the embarrassment of going on national TV!

One problem, I find, is that many of the letters I get are from followers of a whole range of 'alternative therapies'. Although these are mostly sincere offers of help, they show an overwhelming misunderstanding of Alzheimer's disease, its causes, effects and progress, not realising the 'cures' they offer may work for some of the other dementias, but not, unfortunately, for Alzheimer's.

It is clear that a simple description of Alzheimer's disease is needed, what it is, how it affects the brain and thereby the person, and what other dementias there are that can be cured.

A postscript – God works in wondrous ways!

When the team made arrangements to come and film us again in early 1997, Micheline let slip on the phone, when making some arrangements with Mike Munro, that I was experiencing some financial problems at the time. Well, with overwhelming generosity, he later rang Ianthe and said that they would like to bring us a cheque for $1000 as a gift, and would that be OK? That evening I was embarrassed, but pleased to accept this offer.

And then, when I added up all the outstanding bills that I had been accumulating and unable to pay, the total was $999.95! So I joked with my daughter about how the 5¢ would go in the collection plate – but said that although God had certainly provided for us, he should have arranged for $1100, so that there would be 10 per cent left. In the week or so that followed I also began to wonder whether all these companies would wait until the cheque had been cleared.

So I was even more amazed when on the day the film crew came, Ianthe and I were taken aside by Mike and given $1450 in cash – enough to pay my bills (cash, so no clearance time), compensate Ianthe for the day's wages she had foregone to be there for the filming, and $150 left over for the collection plate!

God's very much in charge, and certainly works in mysterious ways!

Chapter 17

Do I really believe in healing?

'I'm planning on writing a book,' I said, somewhat optimistically and overconfidently, to my specialist.

'I'd be very interested to read it,' he said.

'How long will I be able to write? When does that ability get lost?'

'Well, it differs from person to person, but if you want to write, I'd do it as soon as possible,' he answered.

Medically the prognosis is pretty depressing. The first specialist who saw me in May 1995 had said that it would only be about five years before I was 'demented'. The disease is a progressive destruction of the brain, which in younger patients (it's great, at the age of forty-nine, to be called 'younger'!) nine results in death in about six to eight years from diagnosis.

There is no cure or treatment, only the new drug, tacrine (that I am already taking), that may help the remaining brain to work a bit better, but doesn't slow down the damage to the brain.

But this is the worldly view and experience of Alzheimer's. With God all things are possible. Already the damage to my brain, clearly visible on all the scans taken in 1995, is such that I should probably be much more disabled by now. But God is clearly at work in all those empty spaces in my brain – and a miracle is in progress! My brain is finding new ways to use more and more of its reserve, and functioning quite well, despite all the missing bits.

Writing this book about my experiences is yet another triumph of faith over medical expectations – the specialist's advice to write quickly was way back in early 1996. I'm still writing, and planning to write more things for my daughters. Thank God God's in charge! I am sure I can ignore statistics – and doctor's expectations – and focus on being as well as I can, and writing down as much as I can for my girls!

God can, at the very least, heal us from any negative attitudes to our sickness, to take away any fear or depression. At times there is no cure – otherwise no-one would ever die! But whatever the outcome of sickness, our faith does give us joy which is incomprehensible to non-Christians, and a chance to witness to others just how powerful and transforming this living God can be. I am still learning, and know that I must accept healing by faith even if this is not always possible by sight (or evidence about my medical condition). Certainly I have my bad days when I cannot cope with the assault of sight and sound inputs.

But I have many good days too, when I wonder if I am really sick at all! These I treasure, as part of the many blessings given to me and my three girls. I believe there is absolutely no doubt that God is at work in my life, as well as in the lives of Ianthe, Rhiannon and Micheline. I put my faith and trust in this and I know that our church 'family' and friends are an important part of this ongoing blessing.

I have received so many loving, caring phone calls, letters, visits, flowers and hugs from the congregation – which are welcome outward signs of the prayers that I know they continue to offer for my family. My three girls have also received care and nurture from them, and from the Young Disciples group for teens that meets at our church each Friday night, and Camp Pelican, the Anglican diocese holiday camps for primary and secondary school children. It's scary to think how difficult it could have been if I did not have faith, or have that wonderful 'fringe benefit' of faith – my church family!

I feel confident that I am fulfilling God's purpose for me – and that part of this is to write down my experiences for others.

Out of what to others might seem to be a nightmare, faith is doing great things. I must admit though at times I have slipped into a worldly view of fear of the future and anxiety for my girls, and have found that this leads to despair. But my faith keeps me going so that even in times of desperation I have been able to come through with joy.

I do believe in healing, but can't say that I am healed, only that I am being healed and that a miracle is in progress. Already I could be expected to show more disturbing symptoms by now – but I am functioning reasonably well, thanks to God.

I believe we can all be healed, in one or more of three areas – spiritual, emotional and physical – and it may not be instant, but step by step. Often we expect only the outward, physical signs of healing (or 'cure'), but I am finding out that the inward signs are just as, if not more, important. Also we need, I think, to be more attuned to gradual healing. We often get sick bit by bit, so why not get better by tiny, seemingly imperceptible steps?

Many months after writing this, I read Kenyon McKie's *Sermon for Synod Evensong*, 1996. He, too, talks of the difference between a cure (removal of disease) and healing (meaning wholeness of body, mind and spirit), and says that even if we are physically cured, we still need healing.

I have been healed spiritually and emotionally, of the doubt of where God might be in all of this, and of the fear of the disease. This happened in stages.

First I was given great reassurance of God being very much with me in my suffering, when I lay on that scanning table I spoke of before, sick with fear, and had a lovely vision of lying instead on lush green grass, bathed in a radiance I knew was from God. From that moment I have drawn great strength from an inner sense of peace.

Then a month or so later I was feeling quite tired and depressed, while waiting for further test results in 1995. I was experiencing difficulty sleeping, and was having some quite scary dreams. As I drifted off to sleep one night I prayed, pretty briefly because I was tired and feeling low: 'Please give me a peaceful dream, protect me from any darkness, and please give me joy.'

Well, I certainly got what I had asked for! I had an amazing and memorable dream, which I now call my 'joy dream'. I was sitting on a swing, which dangled on two long ropes reaching up into the sky, and each rope had been decorated with flowers. I was swinging just above the tree tops, over a leafy and green parkland, through which paths meandered. People were walking in small groups through this sylvan scene, talking, laughing, debating. I knew that not all were Christians, so I was singing at the top of my voice (luckily in my dreams I can actually sing!) 'Jesus, precious Jesus'. I was full to bursting with joy, and wanted everyone down there to share it.

I woke up singing, filled with incredible happiness – it more than sustained me through finding out that the final tests confirmed the earlier diagnosis of Alzheimer's – and that joy has bubbled away there ever since.

Then the prayers of my church for me, and the faith so evident in those around me, enabled me to step forward for healing at a Cursillo healing service in October 1995. Importantly, God used this step of faith on my part to take away all of my fear, as well as my pride (in my intellect, ironically enough!), so I could shrug off all worries and anxiety, and be at peace.

From that moment fear has been easy to cast off, as long as I keep my focus on God. But I sink rapidly if I turn away. I have had to learn this lesson repeatedly, though. For example, I can become quite sick with migraines if I busy myself unnecessarily, and forget what is really important in my life. My hallucinations brought about a real feeling of terror in me, too. But if I am obedient and do what I think God wants me to do (like write this book for instance), then I am never ill – no matter how difficult or stressful the task.

So I do claim quite confidently that I have been and am being healed, spiritually and emotionally. And maybe I will be healed physically too – and that truly would be a miracle, as unlike cancer, I have never heard of any remissions or cures for this disease. For me an eternal perspective on healing is my hope and strength. Even if I will not be physically healed I know that I will be given the strength, peace and joy throughout, to cope with whatever lies ahead. I believe in a God of surprises and it's more a matter of saying 'watch this space'.

A postscript
– a God of
surprises!

Chapter 18

I'm getting better!

Ianthe was busy making the tea, while I stood opposite her at the kitchen counter, bubbling over with the news I had hardly dared to tell her.

'I'm getting better!'

She raised an eyebrow. 'Yes, Mum', she said, in that tone of voice she uses when she is humouring me.

'No. I'm really feeling a lot better. I'm less foggy in the head, and I can get words out a lot easier. It's not all so much effort as before.'

Disbelief was clearly written all over her face. 'Mum's really losing it now,' she was thinking. 'Is this just another stage of dementia? Who gets better from Alzheimer's!'

'I think I'd like to try driving the car again. Only just around locally, of course.' I was in full swing, once I had got over the first step of voicing out loud what I had been feeling for some weeks.

Poor Ianthe! Alarm bells were now ringing loud and clear! You could see a myriad of thoughts flitting through her mind, as she desperately tried to think of a way to deal with this. 'We'll see,' she said, resorting to the phrase I had used so often as a mum to buy myself time in response to the girls' requests. How the tables had turned!

That was in July 1997, and over the next few months we began slowly to adjust to the thought that maybe, just maybe, I might really stop getting worse, that I might even continue to improve, and may indeed be able to function independently reasonably well.

What a miracle!

Mind you, there have been so many prayers for my healing. Maybe sometimes we don't really expect results. Are we attuned to those tiny steps of healing – the gradual getting better? We accept that a course of tablets can take some time to work – why can't we believe God does it that way too?

The girls and I are taking each day as it comes. It's hard to adjust, when over the last year or so we have made plans based on the standard medical expectations. What do we do, now that God has 'put a spanner in the works'? Should Ianthe finish her degree, can I manage alone …?

But all these decisions will unfold easily before us, I'm sure. It's best just to hang on tight to that roller-coaster cart of faith!

Chapter 19

A 'miracle cure'?

It's now February 1998, and I continue to improve. I have been driving, my head remains clear, and I am able to tackle things I could never have dreamed of doing a year or so ago.

It seems as if I have regained a lost year or so in this disease. Although I am not back to where I was when I was well and at work – or even the time when I was first tested for the signs of the disease – at least I am now able to function really well within my own limits, around the home and garden, without any external pressures and demands that can confuse and disorient me.

Some days though, are a battle, a struggle. I am consciously trying to remain alert, to keep my brain active, to try to register things happening and said around me. And sometimes I cover up for the fact that I am simply not really following properly what is going on around me. It takes time to register what you say, as sometimes the words seem meaningless and only sort themselves out later in the context of what you are saying. I am getting so good at covering up, though, that no-one notices!

Occasionally this daily struggle is a bit too much and I get a migraine – but even this is worth being there for my girls – not letting myself slide away into the confusion and abstraction of Alzheimer's.

Obviously I am not always quite 'normal', and sometimes there are total holes in my ability to register things said or happening around me. An example was the time Micheline and I sorted out money for her to go to the shop and buy bread. She then popped upstairs to get her shoes and I sat down on the lounge. As she came down past me and out towards the back door, saying 'See you soon,' I asked 'Where are you going?' I do this sort of thing most days! But I am sure it is very good for developing qualities such as patience in my daughters!

Of course, with those outside the family I'd never ask 'where are you going?', as it is obvious from your tone of voice that I am meant to know. I'd say nothing and wait till you reappeared, and try to work out then what I missed.

And then there are those things I don't even tell my girls – like the difficulty I have sometimes walking on clearly patterned floors, as my perception of distance, periphery and so on relies so much on familiarity and the presence of the usual clues to my environment. Something new can throw me. So I'll stumble over a smooth but patterned floor, or be very confused and indeed lost by changes at my local shopping centre, or by coming in somewhere familiar through an unfamiliar entrance.

But maybe I'm just adjusting well to coping with this disability, and have really accepted my future, no matter what it may be. My faith has given me so much joy it is hard to be anything but positive, looking forward to each day with enthusiasm and excitement. I've become used to the types of problems I have, and have found ways to deal with them in my familiar and quiet environment at home.

I was feeling so much better already, by October 1997, that I invited Anita, a good friend from Germany, and her travelling companion, Wilma, who were in Australia, to stay for the weekend, and even collected them on Friday afternoon from the airport – although baggage collection noise and bustle defeated me and Micheline took over!

It was a beautiful late spring day – a balmy sunny blue sky, fresh new green leaves on the trees, and a painter's palette of parrots and rosellas to show off to my guests. After getting back from the airport, we went out into my little garden, to share a pot of tea – and of course to enthuse over the profusion of colour in plants and birds.

The phone rang and I ran back inside to answer it. It was my mother ringing from England, distraught and hardly able to speak – my father had died unexpectedly that night. My reactions were slow and confused, and my sorrow very deep. Words failed me, tears and hugs are so hard to share over the phone. I longed to be there immediately, to put my arms around her and to grieve together.

My father had been so well, and took his responsibilities of caring for my mother very seriously. She is quite unwell with a number of serious illnesses. His death was totally unexpected.

One great source of comfort for me, though, was that a month or so before he died, my father had read the draft of this book, and had 'heard' me speak out about the really important things in life, and also how much better I was feeling. He was keen to speak to me, too, after reading it. He was always a man of few words, very reticent about revealing his feelings, but the tone of his voice on the phone (and the very fact that he had read every word, although not usually a keen reader) as he said that he 'just wanted to hear my voice' meant a great deal to me. I am really looking forward to seeing him again in heaven.

Ianthe was able to take over that Friday evening, and the whole of Saturday, playing host to our guests, while I gathered my strength. I was determined to go to England for the funeral, and to leave with Ianthe on Monday. Whilst Ianthe organised the tickets, Anita, Wilma and I went to church on Sunday morning, and my church family gathered to send me off with a good dose of prayer.

All my family were concerned about the effect my father's death and the long trip might have on me – but when I arrived they were amazed at the obvious improvement in me since my last visit the year before.

My aunt asked 'What tablets are you taking?' as she saw me regularly taking my daily dose of 2000 IU vitamin E, 2400 mg lecithin and 1g vitamin C. I told her about the ongoing research on vitamin E, but stressed that my main improvement had been after prayer, not tablets.

She was greatly impressed with the change that she saw in me, and wanted to try these 'get smarter' tablets straightaway, as she had been concerned for some time about her memory problems. She bought a large jar of vitamin E tablets and began taking them that very day. 'The tablets will not be much good without the prayer, too,' I said, wagging my finger at her authoritatively.

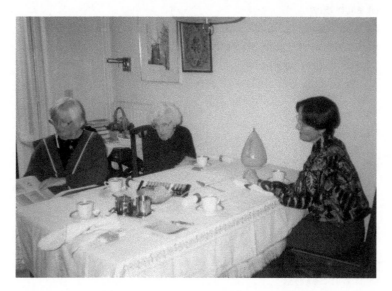

Christine in Antwerp in 1997 with grandmother (then aged 102) and aunt

It's funny how we seem to find it so easy to put our trust in pills rather than in God. My doctors certainly see no harm in my taking the tablets, but they would never claim any of them were the 'miracle cure' for Alzheimer's. Even the tacrine I take (a prescribed medicine) only works in some patients, and they don't know why. The work on the role of vitamins in Alzheimer's is also in its very early stages.

But the fact that I do take vitamins is just the sort of thing to attract interest in those desperate for the 'miracle cure'.

The only 'miracle cure' I can claim is God – and even then I don't have a formula – faith simply doesn't work like that!

Who knows how long this improvement in my functioning will last? The doctors have no idea. Why is it that some sufferers decline more rapidly than others, why is it that some appear to plateau out for greatly varying periods of time? Will my sense of wellbeing last weeks, months, years? No-one knows, but I will make the most of this reprieve to appreciate the true value of each day.

Obviously I will take advantage of whatever current medicine and medical research offers, but I put my trust and faith in God. I have made that choice.

Who will you choose to rely on?

Thank God
God's in
charge!

Chapter 20

Getting onto 'God's roller-coaster'

The phone rang – it was Karen calling from Sydney, in early December 1990. Only a few weeks earlier I had moved to Canberra to start a new job, in charge of a division in the Prime Minister's Department that advised him on science and technology. 'How are things?' Karen asked.

'Oh, absolutely fantastic – life is just so wonderful, I'm so happy, I'm feeling on top of the world!' I enthused.

'Wow! Is the job as good as that?'

'Oh no! – I'm not talking about the job – I've been reading that Bible you gave me, and I've visited Ianthe's church, and… thank you so much, I am really enjoying the New Testament. The job's OK. Yes, it's really good, but I hadn't realised how happy I could be!'

Karen said, 'Praise God! You're my first!'

'First what?'

'First that I've led to the Lord.'

Little did we both know then just how much I would need this new faith in the years ahead, and that I had got onto 'God's roller-coaster' just in time. My faith is like the roller-coaster cart, hanging firmly onto the rails through all of the ups, downs and loops of the roller-coaster ride of my life.

Just try to imagine, even if you are not a Christian, how I (not you – I'm sure you are probably much stronger than me and don't need a 'crutch' like God!) could possibly cope with this disease, robbing me of what had been always so important to me – my intellect – without my faith in God.

So, how did I become a Christian? How on earth did I 'get religion', as I used to be a very busy, very career-oriented 'normal' (i.e. non-Christian) person?

Up to that turning point in 1990, my life used to be an empty 'busyness', with work, studying and family. I was far too busy to find out anything about what I used to call 'that God business'. A relationship with a living God and the strength of Christian fellowship were unknown to me. Church was simply a clique to which I didn't belong and couldn't identify with. Little did I know back then just how eventful and exhilarating life was to become when I finally became a Christian.

My family origins were a mix of Calvinist, Methodist and Catholic. My only contact with church was to be christened in the Dutch Reformed church, going to Sunday school at the local Baptist church because my best friend went there, and doing Scripture at school. My impressions were of all this being a history lesson, not a 'here and now' experience that changes lives.

I started searching for a reason to life in my late teens, impressed by the wonderful design and planning so evident in nature, which is even more amazing when studied at the cellular and molecular level. I tried finding out about Jehovah's Witnesses for a year or so, not realising that this religion is not what I would now call Christian. Then in my early twenties I tried some marijuana, read a few books on existentialism, Buddhism and so on, and tried a bit of yoga and meditation. I found no answer in any of these non-Christian inward-directed searches for meaning.

When I came to Australia in my mid-twenties I was still drifting, looking for a meaning in life, but met my husband-to-be and became pregnant within only a year of arriving in the country. I filled my life with being busy as a breadwinner and mother – as well as surviving life as a 'battered wife'. There was still something big missing in my life, which I tried to fill with work and study.

I believe now that God has a plan for each of us. Other people and events can help us get to a point where we realise what we are being offered and can make a choice to accept God in our lives.

My becoming a Christian was an instant event, but was preceded by what at first seemed to be a string of coincidences, but that now I see as pieces of a puzzle patiently being put together over some five years – to be 'God-incidences', with purpose and meaning.

First I realised exactly what was missing in me when I read a textbook for my Master of Business Administration studies, which spoke of people having three parts: physical, emotional and spiritual. I knew straightaway that a third of me, my spiritual side, was missing, but I told myself I was far too busy to do anything about it.

Then when she was fourteen, Ianthe became a Christian through friends at school. She was the one rescued first in our family – I suppose because she needed God most at that time. She had been deeply unhappy and rebellious for years, and had a difficult and abusive relationship with her father. When she told me about her decision to become a Christian she said, 'I have at last found a real father!'

She became a new person, full of life and joy, and at peace with herself and others. She studied the Bible, stuck 'Jesus loves me' stickers on all her school things – a bit 'over the top' I thought at the time, but it was worth it to see such a change in her. Without her faith, it could have been very different – she might even have ended up on the streets of Sydney.

Also I found out that my secretary at that time was a Christian. She, like my daughter, didn't fit my stereotype of a Christian, or rather a 'church-goer' – and she seemed to have lots of fun!

Later that same year I hired a management consultant to assist in running several planning workshops. Over the holiday break he suggested I read a couple of books. Assuming they would provide some management insights, I dutifully read them. They were *The Road Less Travelled* and *People of the Lie*, which opened my eyes to the reality of a spiritual world and the power of Christianity. I found out that the management consultant was a committed Christian, and Baptist lay preacher. Again he didn't fit my stereotype, he was a highly paid consultant driving a luxury car.

That Christmas I was given a book by my sister who lived in Hong Kong at the time. It was about the walled city in Hong Kong – and unknown, I'm sure, to my sister, it was mostly about the work of Jackie Pullinger saving drug addicts through prayer and faith. Again the power and reality of a Christian faith were shown to me, but still I was far too busy studying for my Master of Business Administration, and travelling a great deal with my work.

The following year, 1990, my new secretary – a 'temp' who only agreed to work for me for a very short period, because she knew I was a demanding career-driven boss, also turned out to be a Christian. She was another challenge to my stereotype. She had a lovely sense of humour, was very good at her job, and didn't (like me) suffer fools very gladly. This temp was Karen, now my closest friend!

At this point Ianthe said, 'Don't you think God is trying to tell you something, placing all these Christians around you?' I shrugged this off as a plain coincidence. But Karen wasn't going to let me get away with it quite so easily. She talked about God, prayer and so on, just in the course of normal conversation, and then gave me a poem that could have been written for me. It was 'The Hound of Heaven', about God following us down all the walkways of life, reaching out to us in numerous ways. Yet again I gave my stock answer – I was too busy to find out about this 'God-business', it would have to wait until I had finished my studies the following year. Karen said, cryptically, 'God might not wait that long.'

I got the message a few weeks later, when (although a very frequent national and international flier) I had a really scary ride on a small plane through some quite extraordinary turbulence on a short, often commuted trip between Canberra and Sydney. For the first time in some twenty years I prayed: 'God, if you get me out of this, I promise I will find out more about you.' Well, we landed safely, and I put thoughts of God aside to get on with work, as I was trying to get everything finished so I could take up a new and even more demanding job the following week – and move house to Canberra over the weekend.

Two days after this memorable flight I went to a farewell lunch with Karen, in a peaceful restaurant overlooking one of Sydney's delightful water views. She had (as she told me later) been in a Christian bookshop when she felt God telling her quite firmly to buy me a Bible. She argued: 'You've got to be joking! How could I ever give such a determined career woman – who drives her staff into the ground – a Bible, for goodness' sake!' But in the end she gave in.

Karen gave me two presents, carefully labelled as 'food for the body' (a large bar of chocolate, for a committed 'chocoholic'), and 'food for the soul' (a Bible). Well, I hugged her, absolutely speechless at how quickly I had been taken up on my promise – my spiritual journey certainly wasn't going to wait until I was any less busy, it was obviously now or never.

The next evening, on the 17th of November 1990 (a date fixed in my memory), after reading some of my brand-new Bible, I went to Ianthe's room and told her what had happened. I had no idea how to go about becoming a Christian, nor any idea what it meant or it felt like. She prayed a very simple prayer with me, inviting Jesus to come into my life.

Immediately there was a change. I felt filled to overflowing with joy and peace, and a tremendous sense of sorrow at having taken so long to turn around to receive all this love. All I could see for quite some time was an intense golden light surrounding me. Jesus in me was unmistakable and like nothing I had ever experienced before. It really was instant – like the instructions 'Just add water and stir', I had simply let Ianthe pray a few words for me, and believed them.

I was a new person, full to bursting with happiness, with love, and – surprisingly for me – with tears. In fact I wept most of the next month or so, whenever I spent time alone thinking about God. Of course, I didn't do anything embarrassing like break down at work, but sometimes it was difficult just to feel 'normal' in the office, when I was so different on the inside, bubbling over with happiness.

Karen's Bible gift came alive with new meaning. I couldn't put it down! Previously, when travelling and staying at motels, I'd pick up the Gideon's Bible whenever I'd forgotten to bring a book. But the words were lifeless, dead, just stories with no meaning for me today. Now the pages seemed to leap out with messages relevant to my life each day, keeping me interested and enthralled.

When Ianthe took me a few weeks later to her church in Sydney, my first encounter with such a supposedly august body in several decades, it was an awesome experience. And there I was, weeping silently with joy and sorrow.

A month or so later I finally started going to the Anglican church in my new city of Canberra. I was quite awkward at first, with the formality of some parts of the service and in my total ignorance of all things spiritual and Christian. I was warmly drawn into fellowship with some of the loveliest people I have ever met, and sensed the very real presence of God in the church.

I realise now just how much I needed my faith. Before, my pride – 'I can do it all by myself, I don't need help' – got in the way of everything. As a child, my nickname was 'I can do it!', and I never really changed that much as I grew older, maybe only becoming even more determined to achieve. I drove myself relentlessly, drove others too, and had a very limited enjoyment of life and all that it has to offer.

Becoming a Christian meant that I had a very real and living faith to help me change gradually from the inside out, and to be more open to others, to life, and to learn gradually how to trust, to let God be in charge of my life. Mind you, this has been one of the most difficult lessons for me to learn.

Chapter 21

Why me – and why Alzheimer's, God?

When I first became a Christian, I was too apprehensive to ask what my future might be, worried that I might not be able to do – or, to be honest, want to do – whatever it turned out to be. Then at last I plucked up courage to ask…and nothing happened at first, just a feeling of a thick grey fog ahead, not knowing what was in store for me.

Looking back now, I'm so glad I didn't know – how much I would have worried, and been unable to cope with the thought of having Alzheimer's disease.

I think of God as the master jigsaw puzzler – putting together a beautiful picture out of so many broken pieces of life, so many seemingly unconnected and upsetting events. I am continually amazed by the way God works in our lives, how – whenever there is a particular problem or concern – there is always an answer, a clear and succinct message always fitting the circumstance. This could be in a sermon, in what my friends say, in what I happen to read in the Bible, God's guidebook to daily living, in what happens around me, or even in a quiet but firm thought coming into my mind, addressing me as 'Christine'. I assume this is from God, as, despite having a 'dementing illness', I'm still not in the habit of talking to myself in that way!

By about 1992, asking God again what his purpose was for me, that grey fog ahead seemed to lift a bit, and I had an inner-voice-type answer: 'Wait awhile and I will call you to my purposes for which you are being broken, made whole and washed clean in my sight.' I even wrote it down in the column of my Bible study book at the time (and had no idea where those words came from). They certainly didn't sound like they came from me. I didn't want to be broken. Scary!

A year or so later I was none the wiser. Here I was, with a successful career, but what did God want me to do? Be a missionary? A priest? A vocal witness in the Public Service? I prayed for months about this, and then in early March 1995 – before I had any inkling of being seriously ill – I got another surprising inner-voice-type answer: 'Christine, you are to be the mother of your three daughters.' That was not what I had expected at all! But I kept praying – surely he had something else as well in mind for me. I was still not really ready just to trust.

By now it was April 1995, and as you know I was seeing the doctor regularly about my debilitating weekly migraines. The phone rang. It was Peta, who had been on a team leading the Anglican Cursillo weekend I had attended the previous year: 'Would you like to be on a team preparing a Cursillo for October? I'll be the Lay Director. It'll involve team meetings every month, as well as lots of prayer, and preparing and giving a talk.'

I was excited, as I had really enjoyed the Cursillo experience of prayer and praise. But could I really do this? I was so busy at work, so sick all the time, and we still hadn't found a way to stop my migraines. Well, as far as I could see, God would have to work a miracle if I was (a) going to be well enough to do it, and (b) going to have the time to put into it.

So I said, 'I'd really like to, but I'll pray about it first and get back to you.' I asked my friends Maureen and Clare to pray about this over the next few days. They both rang back, and Maureen described an inspiring vision involving a butterfly, the symbol of Cursillo. They both felt I should be on that team. My own prayers had come up with 'Trust in me, I *am* a God of miracles'.

I rang Peta and said yes, I'd be on team. 'It's a step of faith, because I'm so busy and so sick, but it does seem as if I am meant to do this.' I wrote in my little notebook (a few weeks *before* the diagnosis of Alzheimer's disease):

By his stripes I am healed. Lord, I must claim your promise to me and not be doubting. The butterfly in Maureen's vision coming from my head is your sign of my release from migraine, your sign that my step in faith is to agree to go on team and to trust in your promises.

The diagnosis, and being told to take six months' sick leave while further tests were done to confirm the diagnosis, were truly a 'godsend'. There was the miracle – time to prepare for the Cursillo, and some relief from my busy life. And then it dawned on me that there also was the explanation of God's purpose for me – to be a mother to my daughters. I wouldn't be doing much else, would I?

Then, over the next six months or so, it became very clear to me what my purpose was now going to be: to try to write down my experiences, not just about me and my girls, but also to explain Alzheimer's in a way that lots of people might be able to understand this physical disease, which whittles away at the brain until eventually life ceases.

Over the years since getting a degree in biochemistry and working for a short while in a research laboratory, I have worked in publishing, writing science in such a way as to be understandable to the ordinary reader. I then worked as an information officer in CSIRO, explaining seemingly complicated research in terms able to be understood by both the public and industry.

And more recently, as I became more involved in the administration and policy side of science, my task was to explain challenging things in writing and orally to very busy ministers, industry managers, and even prime ministers. So I had quite a chuckle when it became clear to me that during my whole career, God seemed to have been training me to write this book!

I am certain that God has a sense of humour – look at the many curious sights in nature. Who could have dreamt up the giraffe, the duck-billed platypus or the crab, but someone with a sense of fun? It did occur to me last year that getting Alzheimer's disease, when I was overly proud of my intellect, could have been a masterstroke of God's irony and humour! After years of thriving on intellectual challenges, of learning new things, of achieving change, of looking down on those at work who were not as quick in their brain gymnastics, now I have been humbled, and realise just how valueless intellect really is.

Looking back on my participation in that team preparing for the Cursillo in October 1995, I can certainly see how much of a strain it was, given that the preparation took place during the six months of tests leading to the final diagnosis. However, despite this, I was still able to participate fully in the Cursillo, and miraculously lasted for four intensive days of group discussion and socialising, without getting a migraine.

It also resulted in an important 'God-incidence' for me – I got to know Liz MacKinlay, the priest on the team, who is also a nurse, and a specialist lecturer in gerontological nursing. Liz was able to give me great comfort during that very difficult time just after I received the final diagnosis and was trying to come to terms with it.

I shared with her one of my main worries at the time – that I would lose my awareness of God before I die. She reassured me that, for those Christians with Alzheimer's whom she has nursed, the one thing that remains in their awareness right to their death is their spirituality. They show signs of being aware of God's presence, responding in some way to prayer and aspects of worship.

I was anxious on the last evening of the Cursillo weekend, when we were all saying our goodbyes, because I was trying to pluck up enough courage to ask her if she'd be my spiritual director. To my delight, she agreed! Liz, of course, is well equipped to deal with my disease, and to encourage me.

We meet now every month or so, and she has also encouraged me to write this book about my experiences of Alzheimer's, interwoven with God and 'God-incidences', which are proving to be such an important part of my life. Without her, you probably wouldn't be reading this, as I would still be procrastinating!

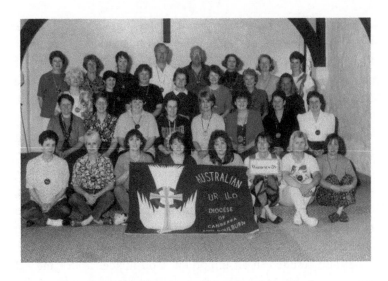

Cursillo Team in 1995; Christine rear row, third
from left, Liz MacKinlay rear row, left

Although I came to know I had to write this book back in early 1996, I made up plenty of excuses as to why I couldn't get around to starting – waiting to settle my retirement from work, getting into a routine, doing all the jobs around the new house etc. Procrastination is something at which I excel! Every time I delayed writing, I got lots of migraines, and very clear inner-voice messages in prayer time, whether I had asked for them or not, about getting back to writing. Every sermon, every Bible study, seemed to talk about obedience. I hardly dared pray, sometimes, because I knew what I would hear!

I was also aware that I might have a biological deadline in front of me – when I finally lose the ability to read and write. I kept thinking that God would make sure I could keep being able to write, until I had finished his work. Or would he? How long could I procrastinate? But whenever I obeyed all this prompting and wrote as much as I could, I never got sick – and my prayer time became much less fraught and guilt-ridden! I found that doing God's will felt a lot better than 'doing my own thing'. There was a lightness, a joy, and a sense of peace.

Writing a book is a good way I can tell people about Alzheimer's, and about God. It's stressful for me to meet new people, and most of my friends are already Christian, and/or know what Alzheimer's is all about now, having seen it first-hand.

Chapter 22

Is God a 'bandaid'?

Liz said, 'It's been a real privilege to share with you this spiritual journey you have made over the last year or so. It's very much like the road I see travelled by much older people as they face death.'

'Well, I suppose what I have gone through is similar to what happens to others, later in life – but this may be already my "later in life",' I said. 'But I'm so glad I became a Christian in time to make that journey. What if I was already in the later stages of this disease? What chance would I have had of finding God?'

We hear of 'deathbed conversions' – where people can at last surrender to God, and go in peace. But if you die of Alzheimer's and have not become a Christian well before the disease starts robbing you of your mind, might not this type of conversion (the awareness of and turning towards God) be impossible? Who knows?

In this book I have shared with you some of my experiences of an incurable terminal illness, and the spiritual journey I have made. I have talked frankly about my faith and what it means to me.

I am now writing material for my girls: about our family history, about my early life experiences and about how confused I was in my early twenties, suffering anorexia, and then having a baby with a man who was already married. I am also writing about how domestic violence has affected each of us, and how scary coping with mental illness in someone close to you can be.

Only some of this covers my experiences 'hand in hand' with God. Much of what I have experienced, and through which I have grown enormously as a person, happened without God in my life. I was forty-one years old before I finally stopped long enough to become curious about what Jesus offered. And my life was no better or worse afterwards than before.

It is not as if becoming a Christian immediately makes it all better – like a sort of giant 'bandaid' for all of life's ills. You know: 'Believe in me and have no more problems!' Just imagine if it was like that, think of the motives people would have for becoming Christians, and then what sort of place heaven would be. It would be full of conmen, liars, hypocrites, opportunists (people who only 'get religion' because of short-term (earthly) rather than long-term (eternal) benefits).

Instead, God helps us be truly contented in the middle of suffering; we know that we are loved and that our suffering is shared. We know that, if we accept that Jesus died for us because we can never be perfect, no matter how hard we try, and we are truly sorry for our sins, then we will enter heaven and be without sin, and be truly perfect without further struggle at that time. This is our eternal perspective – a confidence in great things to come, rather than seeing problems solved today.

What I do know, though, is that if I had become a Christian much earlier in life, and was as much changed from the inside out as I am now, then my life would have been very different – maybe not the events themselves, but how I coped with them.

God has not been a 'bandaid' in my illness, but I have been changed enormously through coming to terms with the diagnosis and my new future. I have experienced greater understanding of the Bible, more appreciation of God's love, the acceptance of God's purposes in my life – and this huge spiritual growth over only three years has been a real blessing.

When I reflect on this journey, I can see that I now have so much more trust in God. I've learned to try really hard to believe God's promises deep down inside me and to get rid of lingering traces of doubt.

If you asked me 'If you had a choice, would you prefer to be well again and not have this spiritual growth?' I have no doubts as to my answer: 'Every bit of it has been worth it and I'd rather stay sick and get inevitably sicker than give away all this inner peace and happiness!'

Chapter 23

Am I afraid of dying?

The ultimate twist in the roller-coaster ride of life has to be death.

Many see it as the end. For me, it is the beginning of a life in heaven, when all people will be perfect – even me. No more personal conflicts, no more sadness, no more blame or pain...

So I look forward to death – or at least to what lies just beyond, as I am very apprehensive about the experience itself. In the meantime, I plan to enjoy every drop of life that remains to me. After all, we are all going to die. It is the inevitable outcome of life. But we usually don't know when, and although I know I may have a limited life span, I still won't know exactly when my life is finished, wrapped up and ready to be presented to God to see.

I believe it is a real privilege to have possibly a limited number of years to get my life in order. Even if I may have only 6–8 years left, this is a wonderful opportunity to live each day to the full. Before this blessing of knowing my days are numbered, I hurtled through life, far too busy to spend time on important things that really matter – like my girls, friends and family.

But I may have longer to live than you, the reader. Suppose you are in a car accident tomorrow, will you have done all the things that you really want to do? If you only have this one day left, can you say 'I have done the things I should have done and one day is enough to finish this work'? Can you rest in the knowledge that you understand why you were here, why you lived your life? Can you face death with your mind at peace?

I have had to face all these questions – and yes, I'm not ready either – and yes, I'm terrified of having to account to God for what I have done with my life. But I'm also blessed because I have had to face these things and now have the time to put my life (and my death) on a better footing.

Maybe I'll wake up and find that the diagnosis, the deterioration, and so on, has all just been a bad dream, and that really someone made a mistake and I'm getting better and can go back to work and normal life.

But then, maybe that's what death is really about – waking up in heaven and finding out that all that struggle and suffering we try to enjoy as life was just a bad dream – the 'shadow lands'. I look forward to that day, when there will be no more tears, no more strife, and only inexpressible joy.

Here on earth I believe the choice is pretty clear between good and evil – there is a mix of both around us that we can experience as a taste of what's to come. We can choose eternal joy, but when God has made the choice so obvious to us why are we so reluctant?

However, I have to be realistic about what might face me and my girls in the years ahead. The disease is incurable, so the only medical certainty is that I will continue to get worse. There are no records of any recoveries, any remissions, no gradual recovery of even the smallest capability lost. All that can be expected is a steady, inexorable decline – and this is our possible medical reality. And it is in this reality that God is beside us, supporting, comforting, sharing our tears, and giving us great peace within. But we have already experienced my miraculous improvement – so now we can live beyond medical expectations, trusting in God, with great excitement.

From a worldly perspective we should plan for my death in a few years, maybe 6–8 years, and in even fewer years, maybe 3–5 years, for me needing full nursing care, maybe in a home. It's not inconceivable that in my mid-fifties, there I'll be, amongst the frail and elderly, for the last couple of years before I die.

But I don't believe any of this needs to be depressing, for God is with us and can still give us so much if we are prepared to look for it, to appreciate it.

I want to carry on drinking in the beauty of this world, feel the love of my family and friends, and even if I might not remember these experiences for very long, I still want to have them. Surely remembering an experience doesn't constitute the sole enjoyment of that moment! Ianthe promises me that she will still take me out for walks and drives, hug me, sing to me, even if I might disappoint her by seeming disinterested or unaware I have just had an experience she hoped I would enjoy. I plan to enjoy each and every experience, even though I might not remember them from moment to moment – the experience of each moment will be enough for me. Even, too, if I don't recognise my daughters one day, I know I will still enjoy being with them, because of the lovely people they are. My love for them won't change – only my ability to put a label to their facial features.

I have also asked Ianthe to make sure that I am never subjected to euthanasia, because I believe we don't choose birth, so why should we choose death. But I have also told her that if I am in the last, severe stage, and I happen to get something like pneumonia, I do not want that treated. My girls must be able to have release from their own suffering, and such an illness would be the chance for me and them to accept God's will with peace and joy.

But I'll be in good caring hands, even if I am in a nursing home – God will never give up on me. Most importantly, Ianthe, Rhiannon and Micheline will also be in God's loving care, and a church family will be always there to turn to – whatever denomination, in whatever suburb, city or town.

I keep praying daily for each of them, that God will not let them go. I know that each may have times when they get caught up in the pressures of the world, when it all seems so unfair and God is to blame, and when all they can see is this earthly perspective, with no hope of an eternity beyond. But at the top of my prayer 'wish list' is that each of them draws closer to God, and chooses the joy that faith offers to those who look for it.

Appendix I

What is Alzheimer's disease?

What follows is a very simplistic explanation of what Alzheimer's disease is, and how it affects a person.

I have written this from a personal perspective, hoping that it may help you to understand those struggling with the disease, as well as have some idea what their families, friends and other carers are going through.

Alzheimer's is the most common reason for a person showing symptoms of dementia. Dementia means loss of memory, decreased intellectual function and deterioration of personality. There are up to seventy causes of dementia, Alzheimer's being the most common. It is an actual physical disease of the brain. Put quite simply, the brain is wasting away and losing its functions, resulting in the person's behaviour changing as the Alzheimer's disease progresses.

What is the brain?

Our brain is quite unimpressive-looking, when you think of how important it is to us. It keeps our whole body going, and even more importantly makes us who we are, giving us our memories, our sense of self, and our ability to think and make sense of the world around us.

In describing it, I'll point out the basics, as well as highlight a few bits that are mentioned when describing what goes wrong in Alzheimer's disease. Basically it's about 1.5 kg of pinkish-grey material, which looks a bit like a walnut, having two connected halves. Each half has been folded up or crushed together so that the surface is made about three times bigger. The 'ridges' of these folds are called *gyri*, and the 'valleys' are called *sulci*.

This folded up bit is called the *cerebral cortex*, which is divided up by a few big 'valleys', or sulci, into four parts:

- at the front is the *frontal lobe*, responsible for our ability to plan, organise, develop strategies, sort things out, and give us self-control or our inhibitions, so we behave in a socially acceptable manner.

- then there is the *parietal lobe*, which does the work of recognising objects from different angles, of spatial orientation (map reading, how objects are placed around a room, etc.) and of simple arithmetic.

- next is the *occipital lobe*, which does the work of seeing.

- then finally the *temporal lobe*, which is responsible for us recognising, remembering (and naming) objects or faces, and for us being able to understand or make sense of sounds and language. Within this, you find the *hippocampus*, which is the organising centre for memory, helping us to encode and store memories, and also to retrieve them.

Deep within the brain is a connected group of fluid-filled sacks, called the *ventricles*, which connect with the whole of our spinal cord. The spinal fluid cushions our brain. If we then could zoom in to look at what this pinkish-grey stuff actually is, we would see special nerve cells, called *neurones*, which have a round cell body at one end, with branches reaching into its surroundings. These branches are the *dendrites*, which receive signals from elsewhere – they are the 'inputs' to the nerve cells. Then there is a very long thread running from the cell body, called the *axon*, which ends in a number of branches, called *synapses*, where the cell sends on its message to others.

The way the cells 'talk' to each other is through electrical signals sent down their axons, which are a bit like electrical wiring through the brain. When these axons reach the junction to another cell, or the synapse, the electric signal is converted into a chemical messenger that goes across to the other cell and starts off an electrical signal through that cell. These chemical messengers are called *neurotransmitters*, and are produced by specialised nerve cells deep within the brain.

What happens to the brain in Alzheimer's disease?

When you look with special scanning machines at brains of people who have Alzheimer's, you can see some differences compared to normal brains. The ventricles are bigger and the gyri shrink and the sulci gape wider, so there is less cerebral cortex, especially at the sides, in the temporal lobes. This is what showed up in my X-rays – the shrivelled walnut – and in my MRI, SPECT and PET scans.

But much of what we know about what is happening right inside the brain in Alzheimer's comes from studying the brains of people who had Alzheimer's disease, and have died, and comparing them with brains from normal people.

Something terribly wrong has happened to these diseased brains. There are tangles within the neurones called *neurofibrillary tangles*, throughout the cerebral cortex and in the hippocampus. The neurofilaments, which make up the skeleton of the neurone, become wound around each other like a corkscrew, after some big changes to their metabolism or functioning. Then, as the neurones die out, these tangles are seen to lie free. Although tangles are not only found in the brains of Alzheimer's sufferers, they do seem to contain many of these corkscrew-like structures. But no-one knows yet how and why they develop, and what relationship they have with the disease. As we are born with our full complement of neurones, all this damage is disastrous – we cannot grow new nerve cells to make up for those lost.

There are also lots of *plaques* in the brains of Alzheimer's sufferers, particularly in the cortex and hippocampus. These are spheres which have a core of a substance that is normally produced when proteins are broken down, called *amyloid*. This amyloid core is covered with a mass of dendrite and axon remains, to make up the plaque.

Again, no-one knows much about these plaques, nor about what this amyloid protein is exactly. Also, many normal elderly people have numbers of these plaques in their brain, although Alzheimer's sufferers seem to have a lot more. But it is far from clear how the plaques relate to Alzheimer's disease. It seems as if the nerve cells' dendrites and axons have died, their protein has been broken down to result in this abnormal amyloid, and the remains of the dendrites are left around the core of this breakdown.

Basically, then, in Alzheimer's disease the millions of nerve cells that make the brain able to do all the things that it does are being destroyed. The destruction focuses on the nerve endings and connections between cells, so slowly closing down various functions of the brain. All this destruction is worst in the frontal, parietal and temporal (particularly in the hippocampus) lobes, so the person has difficulties in:

- *planning, organising, sorting, and behaving in a socially acceptable way.*

  (So I could not plan ahead with a simple computer task, where I had to move some blocks out of one tower into another before moving them back again in a different order.)

- *recognising objects from different angles, seeing how objects are placed around a room etc., and simple arithmetic.*

  (I have difficulty in recognising something from an odd angle, as well as with peripheral vision and quickly moving my eyes around to get a big view of what is around me.)

- *recognising, remembering and naming objects or faces, and making sense of sounds and language.*

  (Hence all my problems understanding what people say on the phone and who they are, and remembering the names for things and people.)

- *recording, encoding, storing and retrieving memories.*

(So I 'forget' – or actually never register – that one of my daughters has just brought the milk in.) Also, the nerve cells that produce the special chemical messengers, or neurotransmitters, are also being destroyed, so not only are there fewer nerve cells as the plaques and tangles develop, but also there is a shortage of the chemical messengers needed to send signals from one cell to the next. This loss of neurotransmitters means that even the remaining brain is having difficulty getting its messages through.

The neurotransmitters most affected in Alzheimer's are:

- acetylcholine (ACh), which can be up to 80 per cent reduced in the brain of a person with Alzheimer's (and without it, 'I am absent' in my daughter's words – very vague and disconnected).

- noradrenaline and serotonin, which are generally more reduced in early-onset patients than older ones, and these low levels result in sleep disturbances (it's not surprising, then, that I am having so much difficulty sleeping!) and impaired cognitive processes.

- somatostatin, whose loss affects learning and emotional control (so maybe this is why I can be a bit teary or a bit too 'blank' emotionally).

Let's look more closely at acetylcholine (ACh), as this is the neurotransmitter most affected by Alzheimer's, and the one targeted – and its levels increased – by the drug, tacrine, that I am taking. Acetyl (A) and choline (Ch) are not combined together as ACh at the nerve junction, but exist separately. When a message travels along the nerve axon and reaches the synapse, or gap to the next cell, the A and Ch must be combined into ACh to jump the gap, and take the message to the next cell. The enzyme (or catalyst) that makes this happen, and makes the acetylcholine (ACh), has very low activity as a result of the Alzheimer's disease.

So there is less of the ACh to go across the gap to the next nerve cell.

The receiving mechanism is OK, so whatever ACh there is gets across the gap – but the problem is that there really is so little to start with. In the receiving nerve cell, there is another enzyme that breaks up the ACh again into A and Ch. It is this enzyme – the one that breaks up the ACh again – that tacrine targets, stopping it working so well, to make sure not as much of the ACh is broken down. This means there is more ACh left around in the nerve cell gap to make sure the signal gets across.

So, the tacrine I am taking works by raising the levels of acetylcholine at the nerve junctions in my brain – basically bathing my slowly deteriorating brain cells in at least one of the neurotransmitters in short supply, to get as much function as possible, despite the ongoing physical damage to the nerve cells.

Why does all this brain damage happen?

Basically the answer is: 'We don't know.' There seems to be a whole range of possible causes, and maybe several have to work together before you actually get the disease. For a few rare cases a genetic cause has definitely been found. But for the majority, there is no clear-cut cause for the disease. Research is looking at such things as viruses, inflammatory changes, environmental effects (such as stress, toxins, anti-oxidants and so on), and the interaction between genetics and the environment.

There really seems to be no *single* cause – no easy answer – and so there is no real progress towards treatments of the actual causes, rather than just the symptoms. It's not even known yet if the plaques and tangles so characteristic of the disease are the result or the cause of Alzheimer's. So solutions seem to be a long way off. At present tacrine, and another drug, donepezil, are used to increase the level of acetylcholine and so help what is left of the brain to function as well as possible. They do nothing to stop the loss of nerve cells, the brain damage that affects the person's very being. But I find tacrine makes a huge difference to me.

Without it, my head seems to ache at the front from strain, and I feel very vague and confused, and terribly tired.

A recent study by a highly regarded research group reported the use of vitamin E and/or selegiline to slow down the progress of the disease. It is thought that their anti-oxidant action might work to prevent or slow down the brain damage – but much more research is needed to verify this and to work out what is actually happening in the disease process and what these anti-oxidants then do.

In both studies using tacrine and the recent work on vitamin E, some additional improvements were noted (although not verified) with people also taking lecithin, which is a material used in the manufacture of brain cells. I've now started taking each day vitamin E (2000 IU) and vitamin C (1 g) as anti-oxidants, as well as lecithin (2400 mg), and it does seem as if they have helped a bit, in making me feel a little less foggy in the head. But it really is so hard to know for sure, with something as difficult to measure as my ability to think, my personality, and my emotions. Who knows, though, if these vitamins are stopping the damage? – all I can say is that I hope so. At this stage nothing is known, there are only hypotheses. The search for a real treatment of the brain damage continues. Only further properly conducted scientific trials, like those begun on vitamin E, can be relied upon to give us the certain answers we need.

What happens to the person as the brain damage gets worse?

At first the brain copes, finding new pathways between nerve cells as old ones become damaged, but then it finally uses up this reserve capacity and the person starts to show the beginnings of mental impairment. The damage doesn't just affect memory, but affects every aspect of the person – their intelligence, imagination, communication, emotions, judgement, motivation, behaviour and self-control. The whole personality slowly falls apart, but the person will look physically very well until quite late in the illness.

Eventually Alzheimer's may lead to death, because there is simply not enough brain left to keep the body going (although some sufferers seem to plateau out for very long periods, but no-one knows why). But death is not the thing I dread most. Rather it is the disintegration of the essential 'me', and the fact that later on in the disease I will not be aware I am behaving in a socially unacceptable way, and perhaps embarrassing myself and my family.

There are three stages to the disease, as various brain functions are lost. A simple rule with Alzheimer's sufferers is that what you learned first usually goes last:

- Hypothetically, at about twelve years of age, you probably could have held a job. That ability goes first.

- Then, at about 7–12 years, you could probably manage simple finances. That goes next, in the early stage of the disease. And so on.

- In the last stages, you lose what you learned as a baby and toddler. You lose control of bladder and bowel, saying a few words, walking, sitting up, smiling.

In the first two stages, mild and moderate, the person is said to be 'dementing'. I'm not sure I like that label applied to me, as I feel quite normal, but just have a few difficulties in some things... but that is the terminology. There is a lot of overlap between the stages, and so we may show features of each of the stages. Certainly, I feel as if I am mostly in the early stage, but can relate to quite a lot of things from the moderate stage. The last stage is severe, when the person is 'demented'. That sounds awful!

The following brief summary of these three somewhat overlapping stages comes from the *Helpnotes* from the Alzheimer's Association of NSW. These are written from the point of view of the 'normal' person looking at the Alzheimer's sufferer. So, for the mild to moderate stages, I have tried to explain – from an 'insider's perspective' – why we might appear to be so odd.

All the material I have seen so far (and this is true for publications from all of the support groups in Australia) are written and produced for the carers of the person with Alzheimer's. Unfortunately we actual sufferers of the disease seem to have been forgotten. Maybe people think that we are too far gone to care. But I do care, and so I have tried to write about what it feels like from our point of view.

Stages of Alzheimer's Disease[1]

Stage 1 – Mild (may last 2–4 years)

We need you to be patient and understanding. I'm in this stage when I'm rested and well, and taking tacrine regularly.

- *apathetic, less sparkle*

  because we're not able to follow everything going on around us, and we're worried we might say or do something silly if we have missed what is really happening

- *less interested in hobbies, activities*

  because we get exhausted so easily now, as our brains have to work harder to do what used to be easy

- *unwilling to try new things*

  learning anything new is very difficult, and we need so much repetition from you (the person trying to show us how to do something) that we know we will annoy you

- *unable to adapt to change*

  we get very confused, as our memories of how to do things the 'old' way are firmly fixed in our remaining brain, but something newly learned just keeps being forgotten

- *less able to make decisions or plans*

  you need to be able to hold a lot of thoughts in your mind at once to sort out and decide which decision to make, and

---

1 Adapted from *Helpnotes*, Alzheimer's Association, in italics, with added comments from an 'insider's perspective'.

we can't do this very easily because there is less storage space for ideas

- *slower to grasp complex ideas*

  like making decisions, we run out of storage capacity to take a complex idea in and to understand it properly

- *ready to blame others for 'stealing' misplaced items*

  our memory of recent events is so defective that we honestly think we have put something somewhere, and have absolutely no recollection of what we may actually have done with it, so of course we think you have taken, borrowed or misplaced that thing

- *more self-centred, less concerned with others and their feelings*

  it takes so much energy to make our brain work, and just keeping ourselves going feels like an achievement, and listening to you to find out your needs is stressful as we so often miss what you are telling us and we are worried about making an inappropriate response

- *more forgetful of details of recent events*

  we may simply have failed to register what is happening, as to do just this takes lots of effort on our part, or we have run out of storage space to keep this memory for later recall

- *more likely to repeat themselves, or forget their line of thought*

  we may well forget what we have just said, and often I ask first 'Have I told you this already?', but sometimes I just sound like a cracked record! It takes a huge amount of effort to keep track of what we are saying, and any small interruption usually means 'we lose it'

- *more irritable or upset if they fail at something*

  we know something is wrong with us, although we desperately want to be normal again, and there is so little capacity when we have made an effort to do something, that if we fail, it is so much harder to have the strength left over to 'laugh it off '

- *seeking the familiar, shunning the unfamiliar*

  anything new takes lots of effort, and our minds become very quickly drained, and we are also very anxious not to get lost or to be a failure in something new we might be asked to attempt

Stage 2 – Moderate (may last 2–10 years)

We need even more patience as well as subtle help, but please don't take over. I'm often in this stage when I'm tired or I've forgotten to take my tacrine.

- *need assistance and supervision with tasks*

  we get confused very easily, and often just can't remember something we used to know quite well

- *be very forgetful of recent events…memory for distant past generally seems better, but some details may be forgotten or confused*

  it is hard to be able to register and store new memories, but somehow our old memories are still very much there, and all sorts of things going on around us can trigger recollection of these past events in our lives, and it is so much easier to talk of these than it is to talk of the present, when we have such difficulty in taking everything in as it happens

- *be confused regarding time and place, and time of day…may go out shopping at night*

  I look at my diary several times a day to keep reminding myself what day of the week it is, what month and what year. Although I used to be able to have a sort of background to my thoughts, easily accessible, which knew all this automatically, now there is no space somehow for this daily record, and it takes more effort to keep these things in mind

- *rapidly become lost if in unfamiliar surroundings*

  I panic if I am somewhere unfamiliar to me, and so there is even less chance I can cope, because I have to remember a whole series of things to be able to orient myself, such as which way did I come, and somehow everything looks so very different looking back than going forward

- *forget names of friends or family, or confuse one family member with another*

  I always know who you are, but the name that belongs to you isn't there automatically unless I search for it, and there is no time to do this sometimes, and the label you have has become unattached somehow and I get the names mixed up, but for me it is no longer important that you have a name, only that I know who you are

- *forget saucepans, kettles...may leave stove on*

  yes, we just can't keep all this new information in our sieve-like brains, so I try now to do only one thing at a time and not to become distracted, because the fact I am cooking dinner under the grill will not automatically remain in my mind if I am also boiling something on the stove, or talking to someone

- *wander around streets, perhaps at night; sometimes becoming completely lost*

  this hasn't happened to me yet, but I can understand how this can happen, because if I can suddenly forget how to drive in the space of half an hour, then surely one day I might forget where I am going, where I am or where my home is

- *behave inappropriately, such as going outdoors in sleep wear*

  I am dreading this, and yes, I can see how it might happen as I sometimes simply forget where I am, who I am with, and what we are meant to be doing

- *see or hear things that are not there*

  yes, I did this when I thought the watering system was spurting all over the garden and needed fixing, whereas it was only raining. I find it very hard to recognise noises, and it now takes a conscious effort when I hear something to work out what it is

- *become very repetitive*

  of course we will, when we have forgotten what we just said to you!

- *feel safer at home and avoid visiting places*

  it is not so much feeling safer but avoiding the extra stress of new environments, of lots of sights and sounds around us, and of having to make conversation and answer all those questions, because we just get exhausted – not physically but mentally

- *be neglectful of hygiene or eating (perhaps saying they had a bath or a meal when they have not)*

  we need things to trigger our actions, for we forget the normal run of things, and somehow hunger doesn't register the same to me any more, so I need to make an effort to remember lunch when I am on my own. I'll tell you I had lunch, for I am too ashamed to admit that I forgot. If I forgot to shower I think I'd know from the smell – but maybe that too will happen, although I hope not!

- *become angry, upset or distressed very rapidly*

  I find I have less mental energy to cope with criticism, or others being angry at me, and because I have so little mental resource, I am more emotional than I used to be

Stage 3 – Severe (can last for 3 or more years)

We need total care until we die. Thankfully I'm not here yet, and I'm not sure how I'll communicate with you from an 'insider's perspective', but I'll try!

- *be unable to remember for even a few minutes that they have, for example, just had a meal*
- *lose ability to understand or use speech*
- *be incontinent of urine and/or faeces*
- *show no recognition of friends or relatives*
- *need help with feeding, washing, using the toilet, dressing*
- *take clothes off inappropriately*
- *fail to recognise everyday objects*
- *be disturbed at night*
- *be restless, perhaps looking for a long-dead relative*
- *be aggressive, especially when feeling threatened or closed in*
- *have difficulty walking, eventually perhaps becoming confined to a wheelchair*
- *have uncontrolled movements*
- *eventually become permanently immobile, and confined to bed in final weeks or months, until unconscious, and then die*

How do you know if someone has dementia?

Some of you might be worried now, as to whether you or a friend or relative have the early symptoms of dementia, and whether it is Alzheimer's.

You might, as everyone does, forget things from time to time, but if you had dementia, you'd forget most things most times, and your memory would keep getting worse. Like me, you'd have to work very hard at remembering everything – writing things down, always putting things in the same place, and so on. Basically, memory and other problems are persistent and progressive when you have dementia, and only occasional when you don't. Table 1 (p.161) tries to show the difference between 'normal' forgetfulness and the signs of dementia.

Isn't dementia the same as Alzheimer's – part of getting old?

Dementia is *not* the result of normal ageing – it is the result of a number of conditions, one of which is Alzheimer's. The person with Alzheimer's has lots of plaques and tangles affecting the brain and its functions (not just the memory but a whole lot more). When you get older, but do not have Alzheimer's, you will have just a few plaques and tangles, widely scattered through your brain, which do not much affect your memory or thinking.

Dementia is *not* the same as Alzheimer's – it is a symptom of Alzheimer's, and of a number of other diseases and conditions. In fact there are about seventy causes of dementia, and some people with these symptoms are actually suffering from depression. In fact, often people are misdiagnosed with dementia when instead they are depressed. They can, of course, be treated. The problems will disappear. Table 2 (p.163) gives some of the most common causes of dementia (recognising depression as a cause of pseudo-dementia) and their treatments, if any.

A significant number of cases of dementia are due to vascular, or multi-infarct (lots of mini strokes), dementia. This can be treated to some extent by aspirin or anti-hypertensives to prevent further strokes. The dementia can be stabilised, but often other factors interfere with its control. Quite a few causes of dementia are partly or fully reversible. So it is well worthwhile to see if there is a suitable treatment or cure for the dementia. Don't assume it is Alzheimer's, and that there is nothing you can do. See your doctor if you think that you, or a friend or a relative, may be showing some of the signs of dementia. It may even be depression, and not dementia at all.

This explains why it was so important for my specialist to do lots of tests, to make sure that I didn't have a dementia that could be cured or treated. It also shows why in the past, or even now, people may be diagnosed with Alzheimer's and then be 'miraculously' cured by hormone treatments, better diets and so on.

If you are unlucky enough, like me, to be in the majority of those whose dementia is caused by Alzheimer's, at least you and your family and friends can then make the most of the time left to you. Perhaps, if the disease is still in its early to moderate stages, you could ask your doctor if you can try tacrine or donepazil to see if you can tolerate one of these drugs that enhance the levels of neurotransmitter (there may be some unpleasant side effects), and to see if they help. Tacrine certainly helps me and about two-thirds of people who try it.

If you want to try vitamin E and C, and lecithin, again make sure your doctor is happy with this. You should never assume that vitamins are totally harmless, nor should you spend lots of money on something that may never prove to be of benefit. Make sure you try any treatment, even vitamins, with the same expectations as for other drugs – if there is no improvement over the period that your doctor thinks is reasonable, then maybe something else may need to be tried.

Get in touch with your local Alzheimer's Association. They can provide information, help and support. And do all you can to support research into this disease, as some day I'm sure there will be some form of treatment, if not a cure.

Table 1 Normal forgetfulness and signs of dementia

The problem experienced	'Normal' forgetfulness	Possible dementia
recent loss of memory affecting job	forget assignment, colleague's name, or business phone number, but remember it later	forget these things more often and rarely remember later
difficulty doing some tasks	doing too many things at once so leave carrots on stove and serve at end of meal	prepare meal but forget to serve it, and even forget having made it
problems with language	have trouble finding right word sometimes	forget simple words or say completely wrong words so incomprehensible
forget time and place	forget day of week or destination for a moment	get lost in own street, not knowing where you are, how you got there or how to get back
poor judgement	temporarily forget child you are watching	forget entirely the child in your care
problems with abstract thinking	find balancing your account difficult when more complicated than usual	forget completely what the numbers are and what needs to be done with them
misplacing things	temporarily misplace wallet or keys	put things in inappropriate place, such as wallet in freezer or keys in sugar bowl
changes in moods and behaviour	personality changes slowly over time	become suspicious or fearful, or flat, apathetic and uncommunicative
loss of initiative	tire of housework, business or social life	become very passive and need to be encouraged to become involved

Source: *Is it Alzheimer's? Warning Signs You Should Know*, adapted with permission from the National Alzheimer's Association, USA.

Causes of dementia

Table 2 (p.163) summarises some of the most common causes of dementia.

Isn't Alzheimer's a psychiatric illness?

Generally speaking, psychiatric illness occurs without any damage being able to be seen in the brain, either while scanning while the person is alive, or on autopsy after death. Of course, chemical imbalances may well lead to some forms of psychiatric illness, and these can be assisted with appropriate drugs.

However, Alzheimer's is the result of slow but inexorable physical damage to the brain – and as the brain is increasingly destroyed, so also the person becomes increasingly affected in his or her daily life. There are no drugs that can address any imbalances in a similar manner to some psychiatric illness. You can't 'jolly us out of it'. We can't help what is happening to us, and neither can you. And it may well be a one-way street to death, as eventually there is not enough brain left to manage the normal bodily functions of life. So please don't forget, we are not mad, but sick. But you can help make our lives easier by being patient, by listening, by slowing down, and by helping our carers as much as possible.

Psychiatrists can help a great deal in the management of the sufferer, and in particular in the support of the carer, who may well have difficulty in coping. Some hospital psychiatry departments are at the forefront of Alzheimer's research into both community and patient treatment.

Table 2 Common causes of dementia

Type of damage	Illness	Controllable or reversible	Treatment
Plaques, tangles and less chemical messenger	Alzheimer's	no	tacrine, donepezil
Damage to frontal lobe and amygdaloidal nuclei	Pick's	no	tacrine?
Lack of blood supply	strokes, vascular dementia	can slow progression	aspirin, lower blood pressure
Less chemical messenger (dopamine)	Parkinson's	no	anti-Parkinson's drugs do not help the dementia
Physical damage	normal pressure hydrocephalus punch-drunk tumour	yes yes yes	shunt operation stop boxing surgery
Toxic damage	aluminium alcohol	yes yes if recognised early on	remove the poison stop drinking
Dietary	lack of vitamin B12 or niacin (can occur as result of alcohol excess) hypercalcaemia	yes yes	vitamins less calcium
Disease	Wilson's disease Whipple's disease neurosyphilis hypothyroidism Creutzfeldt–Jakob disease AIDS	yes yes yes yes no no	penicillamine antibiotic antibiotic thyroid treatment none none
Genetic disorder	Huntington's chorea Alzheimer's (rare) Wilson's disease	no as above as above	none as above as above
Psychological disorder	schizophrenia depression*	yes yes	drugs to manage schizophrenia counselling and antidepressants

*Depression produces a pseudo-dementia, because although the behavioural features mimic clinical dementia, they probably do not represent a true loss of cognitive ability.

Source: Adapted from Table 1.5, *Understanding Dementia*, Jacques, Churchill Livingstone, 1992.

Is Alzheimer's really a terminal illness?

Alzheimer's disease is a cause of death – mostly affecting people over the age of sixty-five. As the 'baby-boomers' begin to reach that age in the next ten years, the number of cases of this disease will sky-rocket, and so will the costs of care.

For some reason, it is statistically an even faster killer for those who get it when they are younger than sixty-five, like me. With this so-called early-onset Alzheimer's, there seems to be more temporal lobe damage, so greater language problems (which seems to fit with what I am experiencing).

Also there are more tangles and cell loss, coupled with more severe and widespread reduction in ACh, as well as in other neurotransmitters. So those who get Alzheimer's when they are younger (than sixty-five) may deteriorate faster, as Table 3 (p.165) shows. But given the lack of knowledge about the disease, it is very hard to generalise from statistics alone. Also, you could easily add a couple of years to each of the figures in the table, given today's improved health care, and better diagnostic techniques allowing earlier diagnosis.

Table 3 Statistics on Alzheimer's sufferers

How old you are when you are first diagnosed (years)	Number per hundred Alzheimer's patients who get it at this age (%)	On average how long you will last (years)	Longest recorded years of life after diagnosis*
Up to 44	3	4.5	6.0
45–49	2	6.1	9.9
50–54	5	7.2	12.2
55–59	7	8.5	16.1
60–64	14	8.4	22.2
65–69	19	8.5	18.1
70–74	17	8.4	21.3
75–79	18	6.1	11.9
80–84	10	5.0	13.4
Over 85	5	4.1	8.3

*Based on data from the 1980s and 1990s. With improved care, new drugs and improved and earlier diagnostic techniques these may be understated for today's Alzheimer's cases.

Source: Adapted from *The Vanishing Mind*, Heston & White, W H Freeman & Co, New York, 1991.

Can Alzheimer's be inherited?

In only about 5 per cent of cases can Alzheimer's truly be proved to be completely hereditary – and early-onset cases seem to be more likely to be hereditary.

There has been some research into these types of the disease. One hereditary form of the disease is a genetic mutation on Chromosome 21 – one of the threads of life, or strings of genes that program all our functions. This chromosome is present in triplicate, instead of duplicate, in people with Down's syndrome. If they survive into their forties, people with this syndrome seem to be more likely than others to get Alzheimer's, and have lots of plaques and tangles in their brain. Chromosome 21 is also the thread in each cell which contains the genes that program the way we deal with our amyloid proteins, which, as you might recall, are the breakdown products found in the plaques in the brain of people with Alzheimer's.

Other hereditary forms of the disease have been found to be linked to the so-called 'presenilin' genes on two other threads in our cells: Chromosome 14 and Chromosome 1. It is early days yet, and although there are lots of interesting findings from all the genetic studies, it is important to remember that only a few cases of Alzheimer's can be definitely said to be completely hereditary – and these tend to be the early-onset cases.

The overwhelming majority of cases are late in onset, where there is probably some mix of genetics, risk and the environment at work. An important development in research into this complicated mix of factors was the discovery of a gene on Chromosome 19, which occurs in various forms, and can influence the risk of getting Alzheimer's. If you have one form of the gene you have an increased risk, but you still could live to a ripe old age without developing Alzheimer's.

Research will continue to press on towards a better understanding of just why some people get the disease and others don't. But at present, if your family is not one of the rare cases of completely hereditary Alzheimer's, we can do little more than look at the statistics to get an idea of your chances of getting the disease.

- If your relative got Alzheimer's disease when they were over the age of sixty-five, then there is less cause for concern. Your chance of getting it is only slightly higher than anyone else's.

- If your relative got the disease when they were younger, like me, then your chance of getting Alzheimer's is much higher – about 20–50 per cent.

So my girls (and my sister) have a higher risk of getting the disease than people without any close relatives with Alzheimer's. But as I don't know of anyone else in our family with Alzheimer's disease, I'm not sure I will worry too much about these statistics.

Does a high level of verbal skills help prevent Alzheimer's?

A recent study of a group of nuns has prompted some interest in whether a childhood in which you develop good verbal skills might in some way stave off either the disease itself or its effects. Essays the nuns had written in their early twenties, about their lives before entering the convent, were examined to see the level of verbal skills they showed. The nuns were tested each year for any signs of dementia, and after death their brains were autopsied to look for the telltale plaques and tangles of Alzheimer's.

It was found that the nuns who had been intellectually stimulated as a child – and showed good verbal skills in their essays – showed much fewer signs of the disease on autopsy. They had also shown fewer signs of dementia.

More research is needed to follow up this interesting study – but who really knows? Parents who read to their children, get them interested in TV documentaries, go to libraries, encourage games and puzzles, and talk with their children, might be able to stave off Alzheimer's in some way. Certainly, the first ten years of life are those when the brain is developing its connections, its way of working. Stimulating a child may well ensure the brain is 'well connected' and ready for all eventualities – even Alzheimer's!

Also, it is thought that keeping the mind active through reading, doing puzzles and so on helps people with Alzheimer's. While we can't grow new nerve cells, it may help the cells to find new connections when old ones die. So the brain seems to keep trying to work around the encroaching damage, and to find new ways to do things. I am certainly enjoying the 'brain gym' that my specialist has said is very important for me!

Appendix II

How am I now, after all these years?

My journey with dementia started with a diagnosis of probable Alzheimer's disease, given the amount of brain damage seen on the scans and my reduced functioning. A few years later in 1998, shortly after this book was first published, further scans and tests resulted in the change of this diagnosis to fronto-temporal dementia (FTD). Now, 16 years later (perhaps a record in survival despite very considerable brain damage that continues over the years) the latest diagnosis is a sub-set of FTD: progressive non-fluent aphasia.

What does this mean? Well, I will lose more and more of my ability to find words, to speak or write, and become mute over time. So I plan to do as much as I can, while I can, to help get the message out there for better support and understanding for people with the hundred or so diseases that result in dementia, including Alzheimer's disease and FTD.

Each of these diseases shows up as progressive brain damage – bit by bit, parts of the brain disappear. The symptoms of the disease – and the actual type of dementia diagnosed – depend on which parts are affected. But all of them are fatal, as the brain slowly disappears and is unable to keep the basic bodily functions going. When I wrote this book, at the age of forty-nine, I had been told that perhaps I'd be in a nursing home within three to five years, and dead by around eight to ten years. That was in 1998. It is now 2011, and I am sixty-two, confounding all of those medical expectations.

My most recent scans show considerable brain damage. The doctors, when asked, all say the same thing: if they saw my scans without seeing me, they would not expect to meet someone who could speak, let alone walk and function as well as I am doing. Perhaps they would see someone lying mute in a nursing home bed? Quite a miracle! My Christianity that I speak of in this book has seen me through the valley of the shadow of death, and I feel very blessed to be able to continue in my faith and fellowship. With this special time given to me, I will do my best to speak out for those imprisoned within the walls of dementia, unable to communicate, fearful and confused.

Why can I still speak and function? Is it truly a miracle of God? Medically, the doctors say perhaps it is because I have made so much effort over the years to speak, to write, to travel, and to challenge myself with new things. 'Use it, or lose it,' they say, and now the concept of neuroplasticity is leading to new ideas of how the brain might keep re-wiring as we age. Stroke rehabilitation certainly assumes some re-wiring to enable lost function to be regained. For me, I lose function each week, each month, and must re-wire continually to keep going. These ongoing efforts are certainly very exhausting, but the results are rewarding – as each bit of brain is lost, a remaining part tries to take over. It feels like running up an escalator that's going down – it's hard to keep ahead of the downhill slide, but at least I seem to be slowing down the decline. The escalator down feels like it's going faster and faster, so I am getting much more tired these days and could not do all that I could a few years ago. Some weeks I succumb to yet another migraine, like those I describe in this book. Maybe it's my brain's way of saying 'Slow down!'

My kitchen is still my planning centre, with a whiteboard to tell me what day it is and what is happening today, and a diary on the counter where I can check what I did yesterday or last week and glance at what is coming up over the week or month ahead. And my smartphone helps me with reminders, as well as games to keep my brain challenged! I have taken a few driving tests over the last few years, in order to retain my licence and be able to drive locally during the day, on familiar roads. So I continue with my brain gym, as well as with the 'purr therapy' I speak of – now we have two Siamese cats that help keep me calm when my anxiety threatens to overwhelm me. I continue to take anti-dementia medication – now of course there are several on the market, and tacrine is no longer available. These new ones are much improved with fewer side effects. I am still living my own experiment in dementia – the scientist I left behind so long ago is dimly present as I observe the changes and challenges of each day!

When I began this journey with dementia, I was forty-six – far too young! It was appalling, horrific, to think of a disease associated with the elderly. But now I'm sixty-two, and somehow it seems more appropriate, less alarming, to be living with dementia. It's more 'normal', perhaps, to be at home with my husband, my girls living with their delightful partners visiting occasionally. No longer am I struggling to be a single mother of three young girls, trying to appear normal for their sakes. Yes, I have a fatal disease, so I am dying from dementia, but I am outlasting medical expectations, and have been given many blessings over the years. I hope that I will continue to live to see many more.

Appendix III

Alzheimer's associations and help around the world

The web site for Alzheimer's Disease International has links to associations in many countries around the world, and gives a lot of information that will be of help to people with dementia and their families, as well as professional care-givers.
www.alz.co.uk

My own web site has a few useful links, as well as copies of some of my talks which are freely available to download as PowerPoint files. You can also contact me through this site.
www.christinebryden.com

Bibliography

Advisory Panel on Alzheimer's Disease, 1995, *Report to Congress, Alzheimer's Disease and related dementias: Biomedical update.*

Brochures and fact sheets from the Alzheimer's Association NSW.

Bryden, C, 2005, *Dancing with Dementia*, Jessica Kingsley Publishers.

Davies, R, 1989, *My Journey through Alzheimer's*, Tyndale Scripture Press.

Fraser, M, 1987, *Dementia: Its Nature and Management*, John Wiley and Sons.

Friels McGovin, D, 1993, *Living in the Labyrinth*, Mainsall Press.

Jacques, A, 1992, *Understanding Dementia*, Churchill Livingstone.

Jorm, A, 1997, personal correspondence, comments on my draft Appendix.

Heston, L L and White, J A, 1991, *The Vanishing Mind, A Practical Guide to Alzheimer's Disease and Other Dementias*, W H Freeman and Company.

McKie, K, 1996, *Sermon for Synod Evensong (unpublished).*

Rose, L, 1996, *Show me the way to go home*, Elder Books.

Sano, M, *et al.* 1997, 'A controlled trial of selegiline, alpha-tocopherol, or both as treatment for Alzheimer's disease', *The New England Journal of Medicine*, 336, pp. 1216–22.

Snowdon, D, 1997, 'Linguistic Ability in Early Life and Cognitive Function and Alzheimer's Disease in Late Life', *Journal of the American Medical Association*, 257(7), pp. 528–32.

Wagstaff, A and McTavish, D, 1994, 'Tacrine a review of its Pharmacodynamic and Pharmacokinetic Properties, and Therapeutic Efficacy in Alzheimer's Disease', *Drugs and Aging*, 4(6), pp. 510–40.